Fighting the Pain Resistant Attacker

Fighting drunks, dopers, the deranged and others who tolerate pain

Fighting the Pain Resistant Attacker

Fighting drunks, dopers, the deranged and others who tolerate pain

by

Loren W. Christensen

YMAA Publication Center, Inc.
Wolfeboro, NH USA

YMAA Publication Center, Inc.
PO Box 480
Wolfeboro, NH 03894
800 669-8892 • www.ymaa.com • info@ymaa.com

Paperback ISBN: 9781594394942 (print) • ISBN: 9781594394959 (ebook)

20200330

Publisher's Cataloging in Publication

Christensen, Loren W.
 Fighting the pain resistant attacker : fighting drunks, dopers, the deranged and others who tolerate pain / by Loren W. Christensen.
     p. cm.
 ISBN 9781594394942
 1. Self-defense. 2. Pain. I. Title.
 GV1111.C675 2010
 613.6'6--dc22

                    2016944170

The author and publisher of the material are NOT RESPONSIBLE in any manner whatsoever for any injury that may occur through reading or following the instructions in this manual.

The activities, physical or otherwise, described in this manual may be too strenuous or danger-ous for some people, and the reader(s) should consult a physician before engaging in them.

Warning: While self-defense is legal, fighting is illegal. If you don't know the difference, you'll go to jail because you aren't defending yourself. You are fighting—or worse. Readers are encouraged to be aware of all appropriate local and national laws relating to self-defense, reasonable force, and the use of weaponry, and act in accordance with all applicable laws at all times. Understand that while legal definitions and interpretations are generally uniform, there are small—but very important—differences from state to state and even city to city. To stay out of jail, you need to know these differences. Neither the author nor the publisher assumes any responsibility for the use or misuse of information contained in this book.

Nothing in this document constitutes a legal opinion, nor should any of its contents be treated as such. While the author believes everything herein is accurate, any questions regarding specific self-defense situations, legal liability, and/or interpretation of federal, state, or local laws should always be addressed by an attorney at law.

When it comes to martial arts, self-defense, and related topics, no text, no matter how well written, can substitute for professional, hands-on instruction. **These materials should be used for academic study only.**

Printed in USA.

To Carrie

A true warrior, as tough as any Navy Seal,
Army Special Forces Ranger, or Marine

ACKNOWLEDGEMENTS

A hearty slap on the back to my buddies:

Martial artist and physician, Dr. Matthew Hing, for helping me understand the complexity of the human body.

Martial artist and veteran cop, Steve Holley, for his knowledge, insight and street experience with numerous techniques.

Martial artist and former corrections officer, Rory Miller for his suggestions.

Martial artist and author, Shawn Kovacich, for sharing his street experience.

And a crushing hug to Lisa, for your constant love, support and encouragement.

PHOTOGRAPHERS

Lisa Place
Amy Widmer
David Tankersley

MODELS

Lisa Place
A'lyse Place
Rickie Place
Jace Widmer
Amy Widmer
Tim Storlie
David Tankersley
Loren W. Christensen

Contents

INTRODUCTION

I gripped the sides of my seat as Dan zigzagged our Military Police jeep through choked traffic on our way to check out a large disturbance call involving dozens of people in one of the many bar and brothel sections of Saigon, Vietnam. Such calls were as common as the damnable humidity in a city of millions where American GIs overindulged in alcohol and drugs and fought over pretty girls, where racial tensions split the military, and the threat of snipers, bombings, and rockets was a constant. But there was nothing common about the disturbance call Dan and I were about to confront.

We didn't find a bunch of drunken servicemen tearing up a bar, as was the usual disturbance call, but rather one man, an extraordinarily large, black American soldier, standing in an intersection in the middle of total mayhem. It wasn't a racial incident, as was so common in late 1960s Vietnam, but rather a bloodbath without prejudice. It was a moving image of that Biblical painting where Samson is smashing a thousand Phillistines with the jawbone of an ass. Only this Samson, who was as big as a FedEx truck, was armed with a ball peen hammer; his "Philistines" were people of every color.

Dan and I moved toward Sampson, our hands on our holstered guns, shouting at him to drop his hammer. He ignored us, either because our commands didn't register in his disturbed brain or because he didn't hear us with all the screaming going on. He did look toward us, though his glassy, unfocused eyes seemed to be looking into another galaxy where he had been proclaimed judge and executioner.

Not wanting to draw our weapons because of the crowd, Dan lunged for Sampson's hammer as I simultaneously moved around behind the monster. I stand six feet in Army boots but my head barely reached the mountain range he had for shoulders. He flung Dan off his arm as if the MP were an annoying fly and commenced swinging his hammer at people, oblivious that I was dangling from his back like a guy hanging from the ledge of a building. I tried to take him down backwards with a strong jerk on his shoulders, but he didn't notice.

I was 23 years old the night I found myself hanging from Sampson. I weighed 195 pounds, I'd been lifting weights since I was 13, and I'd trained in the martial arts for several years. If I may boast, I had developed a powerful cross punch that would send even the heaviest hanging bag bucking and twisting. Nonetheless, my punches into Sampson's back muscles didn't slow his hammer action, nor did he even glance in my direction.

My partner again latched onto the giant arm in an effort to slow his jawbone-of-an-ass techniques, but once more he was sent flying. In desperation, I began punching the big man's spine, wailing away with at least a dozen hits, trying desperately to dislodge a few of his vertebrae. He ignored me, and trudged deeper into the panicked crowd with his avenging hammer.

Just as I was thinking that I was close enough to shoot him without hitting anyone else, a third MP burst into my peripheral vision and slammed the side of his Colt .45 semi-auto against Samson's skull, which sent the giant to the asphalt like a 350-pound sack of cement.

Later, as I massaged my sore hand and wrist, I wondered what the heck had happened. I had a history of dropping people with my big punch, both as an MP and in training, but not only did Sampson not fall from my rainstorm of blows, he barely acknowledged that I was in his space. Talk about a direct hit to the ego.

That was my first experience with a person who could tolerate pain. As shall be discussed throughout this book, there are several reasons why some people are this way. In Sampson's case, he was padded with fat and muscle, and he was flying high on drugs. I'm guessing if that slap with the steel gun had hit him in the forehead, cheek or nose it wouldn't have slowed him at all. However, the MP's gun slammed into his temple, possibly injuring the middle meningeal artery, which resulted in his heavy crash to Earth.

There would be other incidents during my MP duty in Vietnam, a place where so many GIs drank hard, consumed copious amounts of drugs, and were bombarded by inner demons created by the horror of war. With the ironic task of keeping the peace in a war zone, my fellow MPs and I found ourselves brawling with these folks nearly every shift. Of course, not everyone under the influence was impervious to pain techniques, but those who were made up for all the relatively easy physical arrests.

Working 14-hour shifts without days off didn't allow time to develop a system for dealing with these people other than to dogpile them with as many MPs available at the moment. While this isn't a bad technique, it's not doable when the situation is one-on-one. One guy makes for a pitiful dogpile.

A year after I got out of the Army, I was patrolling the streets of Portland, Oregon as a city cop. The intensity of the job was considerably less than in a war zone, but there were always people who were mentally ill and violent, people who had intoxicated themselves into violence, people who had worked themselves into a violent rage, and extraordinarily fat or muscular people who were both violent and resistant to the usual control techniques.

Now that I was once again training in the martial arts, teaching defensive tactics to police officers, and getting lots of hands-on experience working the street, I was able to experiment with ways to deal with people who tolerate pain. This book contains many of the techniques and concepts that I've found, and my friends in the martial arts have found, work most of the time. *Most of the time* is the operative phrase here.

As I discuss in the following pages, there are no absolutes in a physical confrontation. Just when you think you have a sure-thing technique, one that makes everyone in your class groan and writhe, you'll run into someone who, for several reasons that are discussed in a moment, shrugs it off. So what do you do then?

Read on…

CHAPTER 1

THE NUTS AND BOLTS
OF FEELING NO PAIN

There is a truth in the world of hand-to-hand combat that too many martial artists aren't aware of or refuse to believe: Every time you discover a sure-thing technique, one that makes all your training partners groan and writhe in agony, there exists out there in the mean streets, a host of people who won't feel it. If you haven't dealt with such a person, understand that the sudden realization that your technique isn't working can create an instant pause in your thinking and in your actions.

Consider what martial artist and author Steven J. Pearlman wrote in his excellent book *The Book of Martial Powers:*

The opponents who challenge us do so first and foremost through a mental action, an act of will or intention. As long as their will remains, we will need to contend with them. We can strike them, lock them, grapple them, shed their blood, and break their bones but if they still possess the will to continue at us, they will do so. In this sense, we apply physical martial arts techniques to their bodies in an effort to reach their minds. We interact with their body-mind through pain, injury, or submission until their body convinces their mind to relent.

Pearlman talks about an attacker's will to continue, even after we *strike them, lock them, grapple them, shed their blood, and break their bones.* Sometimes the attacker's will remains as a result of not feeling the pain from all these things you have done. His brain has blocked the incoming signals. Therefore, you must either change your technique to one that is so painfully acute that it penetrates his dulled brain, or forego pain and opt for a technique that incapacitates his ability to attack you.

CONTROL

Before we examine these people who might be tolerant to pain, let's look at three objectives to keep in mind when dealing with such formidable attackers. In short, your task is to control the violent person, control the situation and control yourself. All three are interrelated because without any one of them, there is no control of the other two.

CONTROL OF THE ATTACKER

Control is established by a strong, confident presence, the application of calming words, control holds, punches, kicks, strikes with environmental objects, or any other technique that incapacitates the person's physical ability to attack.

CONTROL OF THE SITUATION

You control a situation by your confident presence, calming words, use of your surroundings, strategic positioning in relation to the threat, help from a friend, and an understanding of your own physical vulnerability.

CONTROL OF YOUR ACTIONS

Sometimes a defender, out of fear, anger or lack of confidence, will overreact and use more force than a situation requires. So this doesn't happen to you, know that when you're in command of both the situation and the attacker, you're more likely to control yourself, even when you discover that the threat has a high tolerance to pain.

A martial arts friend says, "Fighting is about chaos and your objective is to bring order [control] to it." This objective and mindset must guide your actions so that you do what needs to be done for your safety and with minimum injury to the attacker.

Note: Although many of the techniques in this book are designed to debilitate an assailant who hasn't responded to other control measures, you must always strive to affect minimum injury. It's the legal thing to do and it's the honorable thing to do.

I know I'm preaching to the choir here, and that's okay. We all need to be reminded from time to time of these three control factors since they are never more important than when dealing with a violent person who doesn't react to pain.

It's easy to become conditioned to the way training partners respond to our techniques: their frantic slapping on the mat, the way they cry out in agony, how they clutch desperately to whatever hurts, and their comments about your mother. Your training can so condition you to this that when a street attacker doesn't respond similarly—he only mildly reacts or he doesn't react at all—it can cause that aforementioned physical and mental freeze. It's happened to me and I've seen it happen to others.

WHO ARE WE TAKING ABOUT?

Here are the categories of attackers in which there are always a few who can tolerate pain to some degree.
- Attackers who have large fat or muscle bulk.
- Attackers who are intoxicated on alcohol.
- Attackers who are under the influence of drugs.
- Attackers who are out of control with rage.
- Attackers who are mentally deranged.
- Attackers who feel pain but like it.

PEOPLE WITH EXTREME BULK

People carrying excessive fat or muscle bulk are often tolerant of certain pain techniques simply because their mass prevents proper application, or it literally pads the pain receptors.

On one occasion, several officers and I were dispatched to help an ambulance crew control a 400-pound former Olympic weight lifting competitor they had gotten onto a gurney. The giant man was normally a pleasant fellow but he had run out of pain medication that he was taking for a crushed nerve in his neck. He had dropped a monstrous barbell on his top vertebrae a couple of years earlier.

Our entire encounter lasted about 45 minutes, in which every four or five minutes he would go stark raving mad. One moment he would be chatting pleasantly with us, and the next his face would abruptly scrunch, and he would groan, "Here it comes, boys" a warning that some violent thrashing was about to commence. The situation didn't call for us to hit him with a baton, Taser him, or apply a pain constraint hold, which he wouldn't have felt anyway. Nonetheless, when the pain hit, we had to control him for his safety, his mother's, ours, and so he wouldn't damage his house any further.

So we dogpiled him, draping ourselves over his arms, legs and torso (handcuffs were too small for him as were the gurney straps), and then hung on for dear life. Some officers were launched into the air by his massive flailing limbs, while others held on fast to their assigned stations, enjoying a sort of carnival ride until the poor man's 60-second pain surge subsided and he was once again his affable self. During one of the breaks, we secured his arms, legs and huge torso with twisted bed sheets. That enabled us to get him to ER where he received four times the normal dosage of tranquilizers.

This is an example of improvising. We started with a six-man dog pile, which worked for a while, though I don't how much longer we would have tolerated being tossed about. Then we made rope-sheets, which held him fast until we got him to ER.

This big man was lying down the entire time of our contact. What about one who is standing? The hardest part of taking a well-padded and pain-resistant standing person to the ground is unbalancing his large mass and weight. Once that is done, big people usually go down easily because their weight works against them.

Remember the axiom: *Where the head goes the body follows*. With that fighting concept in mind, practice techniques that:
- push the big attacker's chin up and back.
- push the back of his head forward and down.
- take advantage of any weight shift to force the big person down in whatever direction he's leaning.

These concepts are also applicable when dealing with normal sized people who are impervious to pain. You will see these in action throughout this book.

One six-foot four, 230-pound officer told me that he was the lightest of four others who dogpiled a huge man who was violent on PCP. The combined weight of all the officers was well over half a ton, and although at first the big subject could easily move the pile around, they quickly wore him down to a point where they could apply restraints. The officers were aware that the tremendous weight on the man could suffocate him, so once the cuffs and hobbles were on, they got off.

The dogpile is an effective technique as long as you know where the threat's hands are and as long as you don't stay on top of him too long.

Note: Be careful tripping and sweeping big people because it really hurts when they fall on your leg.

PEOPLE INTOXICATED, HIGH, ENRAGED AND MENTALLY ILL

I'm placing these four types into the same group, since the common thread among them is that some people in all four function with a dulled consciousness.

There is a wide-range of responses to pain within this general category. Some feel a little and others feel nothing. Here is an example of someone in the latter group.

A fellow officer got a call on a pregnant woman who had been stabbed in the stomach, the suspect last seen somewhere in the blocks between houses. The officer eventually found the man in a backyard, and ordered him at gunpoint to drop his knife and lie down. Glassy-eyed and either mentally deranged or high on something, the man began slashing the air with the blade as he advanced toward the officer. Not until the officer backed into a garage wall did he fire a .45 caliber slug into the assailant's chest.

As if in a nightmare, the man ignored the hit and continued to slash the air as he advanced toward the officer. With no other choice, the policeman, who was also a member of SWAT, fired a second shot into the man's chest. Again, he only twitched and then continued his advance. So the officer shot a third time, bending the man toward the gaping wound. Again, he straightened and slashed at the officer.

So the cop fired a fourth and fifth time. Only then did the man drop dead into the grass.

Round after round into critical targets and all the subject did was twitch each time he was hit. Do you have a technique that's more powerful than a .45 slug? I don't either.

Pain Receptors

Whether you're applying a wristlock or raking your fingers across an assailant's eyeballs, his brain receives "ouch" signals by a type of pain receptor called nociceptors. Some parts of the human body have many of these, while other parts have only a few. The eye, for example, has more than the chest, wrist or back. Case in point, a person suffering a heart attack complains of a dull ache in the chest while a person whose pointy finger is suddenly wrenched in a direction it isn't supposed to go, screams and utters every blue word in the *Book of Swearing*. (Don't bother looking, it doesn't exist.)

Anytime you deliver force over a relatively large area, a kick to the assailant's back, for example, fewer pain receptors are activated than when you apply that same force to a smaller area, such as a heel kick to his gums. Some people under the influence of alcohol and drugs experience a dulling of the consciousness, and some people in a state of extreme rage or mental illness experience an over-riding of the consciousness. This means that there are some in both groups who might not feel broad-surface pain but will feel acute pain signals.

KEY CONCEPT

Pepper Spray

Regardless of what the ads claim, pepper spray doesn't always work on the street, and never is this truer than when the threat is violent with rage, mental illness, or high on booze or drugs. I've seen sprayed people shake their head like a wet dog and then continue fighting.

Pepper spray is only a tool. Don't count on it as the end-all defense, especially against pain-resistant people.

There is no guarantee when applying pain to a violent person whose mind is altered by one of the mental conditions being discussed here. Additionally, consider that by the time you're forced to defend yourself, the person is likely at the peak of his rage, intoxication, drug high, or psychotic behavior.

What is important when dealing with people impervious to pain is the same thing that is important when dealing with any hostile person: When something isn't working for you, you need to switch tactics. Logical? Not always. Perhaps you've heard the stories of panicked people in a burning building pushing against a locked door over and over until it's too late to take another avenue of escape. The same thing can happen when an adrenaline surge takes over your rational thinking. You hit a violent person, say, in the chest. When that doesn't get the desired effect, you keep hitting him there, over and over. Of course, you might eventually wear the guy down, but since he isn't feeling the blows, the window of opportunity is wide open for him to attack you in some fashion.

PEOPLE WHO LIKE PAIN

There are many reasons why a person will grimace and smile as you give him your best shot. He might be smiling simply because he is drunk or high and doesn't feel it, he might have had a violent past and is conditioned to pain, or it could be some sort of sexual issue with him. It might even be a blend of all these things.

Consider the Groin

When a student gets whacked in the groin in class, he drops into fetal position and begins channeling Nancy Kerrigan: "Whyyyy? Whyyyy?" But in the street, striking an aggressor in the groin gets mixed results. Sometimes he curls to the sidewalk in agony and sometimes he doesn't give the hit a passing thought. The problem is that there is no way to tell by looking at someone as to how he will react to a groin hit.

The groin is a good target; just don't stop to watch for a reaction. It's better to flow into a second, third, or however many techniques it takes to stop the threat.

Does it Work?

TRAIN TO KEEP ATTACKING

It's important to train in such a fashion that you don't become unnerved when someone doesn't react to your best joint lock, palm-heel strike, or roundhouse kick. Here is why. Say you apply a joint lock on a nasty drunk, the same technique that made your classmate dance funny-like on his tiptoes. Not only does the intoxicated man not react, he looks puzzled, as if he isn't sure what you're doing and what you want from him. You look puzzled, too, as you wonder why the technique isn't eliciting the usual yelp and chest slap. Then, because you allowed half a dozen seconds to pass during your confusion, the drunk smashes you in your puzzled face.

When a radio talk show host doesn't say anything for a few seconds, it's known as "dead air," and considered a bad thing. When you pause or hesitate in a physical confrontation while the threat is still, well, a threat, that too can be a bad thing.

To prevent this, you must train physically as well as mentally to keep on the offense until the seemingly invulnerable person is under control. Say you kick the man in the thigh twice, neither blow drawing so much as a grimace. Although you see his lack of reaction, don't pause to wonder what went wrong. Instead, immediately hit targets where there are more pain receptors, targets that shock the brain, or targets where an injury greatly reduces the recipient's ability to attack.

Dealing with any combative person is seldom easy and always dangerous. This truth is magnified many times over when the attacker is impervious to pain, when he neither reacts nor acknowledges your techniques. Happily, you don't run into these types of people often, but when you do, it can be a real challenge.

The following pages present techniques and fighting concepts that have worked for me and for others who have dealt with these formidable people.

When I first began working on this book, I asked a high-ranking jujitsu instructor about the mechanics of a particular technique. He answered my question and then added, "When done correctly, this hurts everyone."

Out of politeness, I didn't respond. But I will here.

No, that technique doesn't hurt everyone. There are people out there who will eat it, smile and keep coming at you. And that is what the rest of this book is about.

CHAPTER 2

BACK OF THE HEAD, TEMPLE, MASTOID AND EARDRUM

I once broke my hand on a guy's head, although he wasn't affected at all. On another occasion, I hit an armed robbery suspect with a no-big-deal snap punch and the blow fractured his cheekbone, released a geyser of blood, and sent him to the ER.

Most readers probably have a story about seeing someone take a head shot only to go on about their business as if nothing happened. Perhaps you have seen a person take a seemingly light hit to the face but go down like the proverbial lead balloon. In the world of MMA fighting, there is always a competitor who gets his nose smeared like jelly on toast but simply shrugs it off. Then there are those pros who bite the canvas after what looked like a light kick to the head, making you wonder if it's a fix.

While we can agree that attacking the head can be unreliable, especially when the recipient isn't receptive to pain, there are some targets there that are more likely to get a response than others. (Look at all the qualifiers in this last sentence: *can be*, *some*, and *more likely*. This is because there are no absolutes when dealing with the human body, especially when its brain isn't receiving pain messages from its parts.)

Warning: Anytime you hit someone in the head, there is a potential for serious injury and death. Not only can the initial target be damaged, the brain is highly susceptible to injury, too. As always, be justified to use these techniques.

BACK OF THE SKULL

EXTERNAL OCCIPITAL PROTUBERANCE

A hard blow to the external occipital protuberance can, depending on its severity and the recipient's vulnerability, stun him so that:

- you can escape.
- you can quickly apply a leverage technique.
- he falls to the ground.

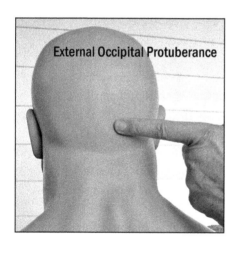

External Occipital Protuberance

In the mid 1960s, I was trying to impress a college girl in class about my karate prowess as a newly ordain green belt. Since karate was still relatively unknown then, she mimicked a knife-hand chop in the air, and asked, "Like this?"

I told her yes, and then in my clumsy teenage way, I knocked all the books off my desk.

The last thing I remember was bending down to pick them up and hearing her again ask," Like this?"

Then my skull exploded, at least it felt like it. There was a moment of blackness, and then a lot of thundering pain in my head as my unfocused eyes and brain struggled to grasp that I was now sprawled on the floor. There was nothing confusing about the girl's giggle, though, and her proclamation of new found power: "That was soooo cool."

Potential Brain Injury

Not only can the boney ridge and the brain tissue directly underneath be damaged from a hard blow, but tissue on the opposite side of the brain can be affected, too. Since the brain is basically suspended in liquid, a blow to the back of the head will send it slamming into the opposite side of the skull.

Dr. Matt Hing, a physician friend and 3rd-degree black belt, explains it like this: "In my opinion, striking the occipital protuberance would stun and cause someone to lose consciousness. Worse, they might suffer bruising and/or bleeding in the brain, which could cause them to go into a coma. They could go blind (the part of the brain that processes vision is right under that occipital protuberance), suffer brain damage (the front of the brain, which analyzes information, can be shoved against the front of the skull), or they could even die. In my opinion, this is a dangerous target for the martial artist who doesn't want to permanently harm an assailant."

Warning: A blow to this target is potentially devastating. Be justified.

CAUTION

When I finally regained my senses, although my head would hurt for a long time afterward, I realized she had chopped my external occipital protuberance. I didn't know its name then (and couldn't have pronounced it given my fogged brain), but I definitely felt where she had hit me. Actually, I knew two things: I knew where she had hit me and I knew that I wanted to slam my desk into her face. I didn't, though. I just moved to a different desk across the room where it was safer. "The art of fighting without fighting," Bruce Lee called it.

On the following pages are a few ways to target the external occipital protuberance.

FACE-TO-FACE CLOSE IN

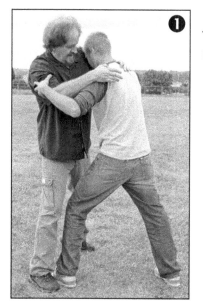

The attacker has pulled you in close. During the scuffle, you free one arm.

Shoot your fist beyond his head...

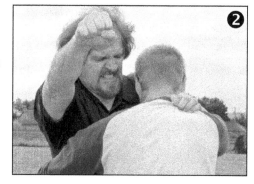

...then snap it back into his boney ridge, striking with the thumb side. With practice, you can generate tremendous force from this seemingly awkward position, even more when you support his head. Hit until he releases, then flee.

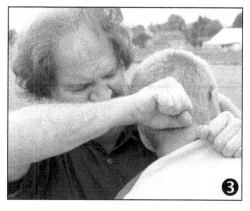

FACE-TO-FACE AT A DISTANCE

When the attacker is at arm's reach, you're going to have to wait until he turns his head to hit him.

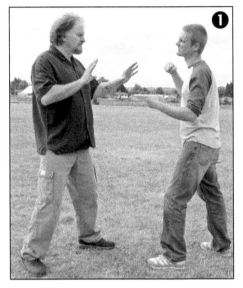

You've been confronted by a mentally deranged assailant and you can't get away. Keep your hands up in a non-threatening posture – although they are in position to go into action – and wait until he...

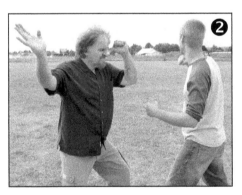

...turns his head to the side. He might be distracted by something or he might be looking at a buddy.

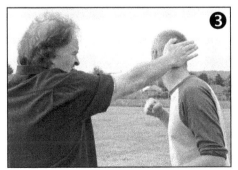

Whip a hard slap against the back of his head, drop-stepping to add power.

FACE-TO-FACE AT A DISTANCE OPTIONS:

Option 1:

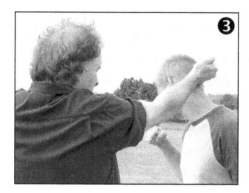

Slam the target with a hammer fist.

Option 2:

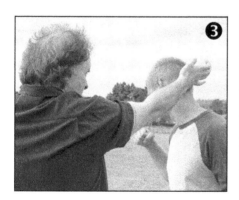

Chop it with a knife hand.

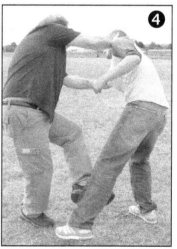

Once he is stunned, take him down in whatever direction he is leaning.

AGAINST A PUSH

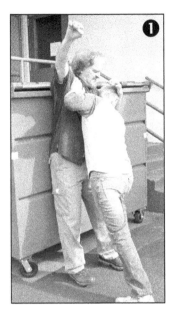

The attacker pushes you against a Dumpster.

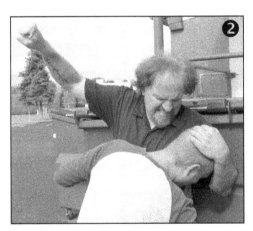

If his head is slightly below yours...

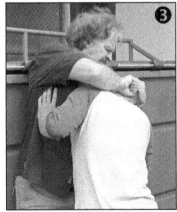

...hit him with the thumb side of your fist.

AGAINST A TACKLE

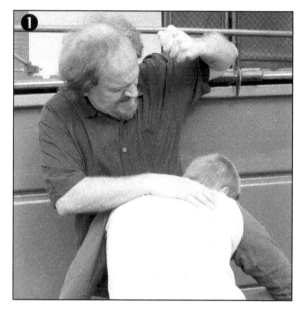

When he tackles you around your legs and his head is relatively low...

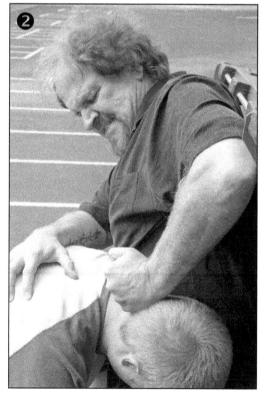

... hit him with the bottom of your fist until he releases his grip. Flee.

ON THE GROUND

You're taking an armed assailant to the ground when, for whatever reason, your technique deteriorates and he begins to get up.

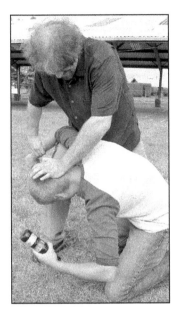

Palm-heel his external occipital protuberance.

Option:

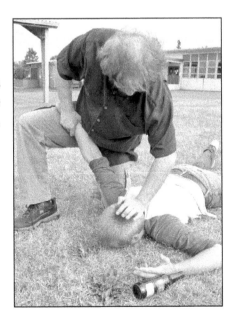

Because the ground is bracing his head, the impact is magnified. Flee.

TEMPLE

Newspaper article, August 17, <u>1884</u>, White Plains, New York - *A few nights ago a fight occurred in a place kept by Mrs. George Reith, next door to the Post Office in White Plains. The participants were Andrew O'Rourke, Edward O'Rourke, and a young man named Joe Acton. They were all more or less under the influence of liquor. Acton got the better of the others and the fight was continued on the street. George W. Potter, an old man of 69 years, kept a restaurant next door to Mrs. Reith. He made some remark against Acton, when the latter attacked him and struck him a violent blow on the left temple, which felled him to the floor. He was picked up in an insensible condition and conveyed to his room. He remained insensible until Friday evening, when he died. A post mortem examination found that the old man had died from congestion of the brain.*

While the 1800-style writing in the above news story makes for a quaint read, it reveals just how easily someone can die from a blow to the temple. More recently, professional boxer Becky Zerlentes died from a punch to hers. The drunken fighters in the news story fought with their hard-knuckled hands, while the pro boxers, who were no doubt in top physical condition, fought with heavily padded gloves.

Do a little research and you'll find many incidents of blows to the temple from fighting, flying baseballs, and falls, that seriously injured or killed the recipients. The temple is a highly-vulnerable area that should be targeted only as a last result.

My friends Lawrence Kane and Kris Wilder discuss the vulnerability of the temple in their excellent book *The Little Black Book of Violence: What Every Young Man Needs to Know About Fighting*, published by YMAA. They write:

The temple is the weakest structural area of the skull where it flattens at the sides, about two-finger-widths back from each eye. The weakness exists because curves are architecturally much stronger than flat surfaces. Shock transmits through the skull most easily at these points. A strong blow to the temple can cause massive hemorrhaging of the meningeal artery, coma, and eventually death. On a lesser scale, a blow there can affect dizziness, confusion and brief unconsciousness.

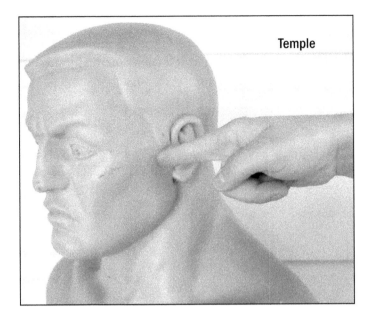

Temple

As with all targets discussed in this book, the objective is not to kill the pain-resistant assailant, but rather to affect some form of mental or physical debilitation so you can escape or follow-up with additional debilitating blows and takedowns.

TACKLE

When you're tackled and going down, slap the attacker's temples before you land. Hitting *as* you fall is counter intuitive so you need to practice to do it under stress.

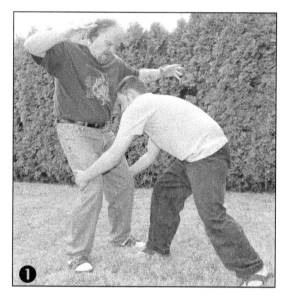

The assailant shoots for your legs.

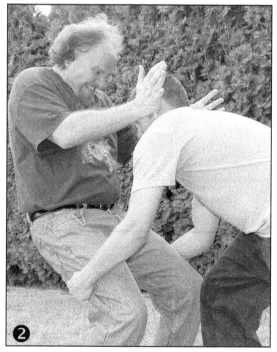

Heel-slap his temple(s) with one or both hands as you fall.

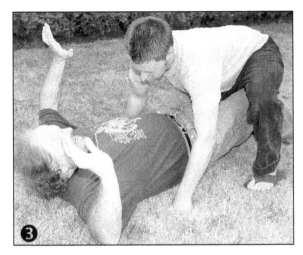

Try...

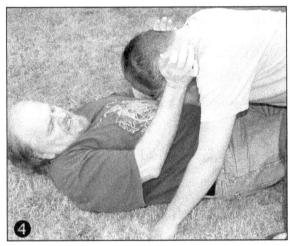

...to hit him again...

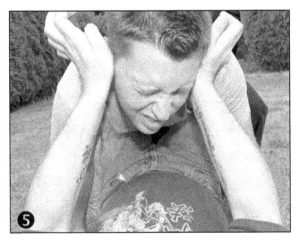

...as you land.

ASSAILANT ON TOP

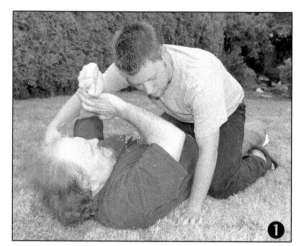

You manage to
block his right
punch.

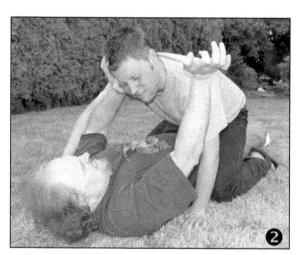

Immobilize his
head, grab the
side of it with your
blocking hand and
then...

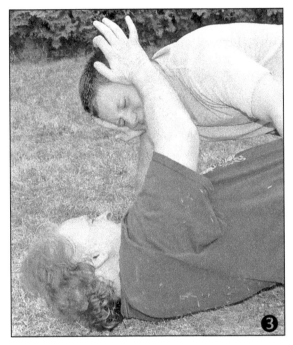

...slam his temple with the heel of your other one. Repeat if needed...

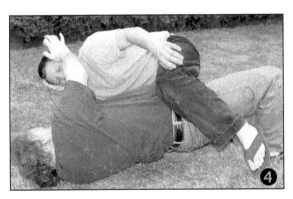

...and buck him off. Get up and flee.

MASTOID

The mastoid is that hard bone where your ear attaches to your head. A blow to it might or might not cause a knockout, but it will likely shock the pain resistant attacker's brain, rattling it enough to make him stagger. Hit it with your fist, palm-heel, knee, shin or instep.

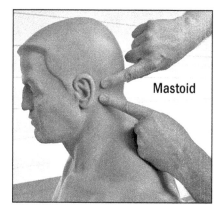

Mastoid

Warning: There is always a risk when striking a bony weapon against a bony target.

KNIFE HAND

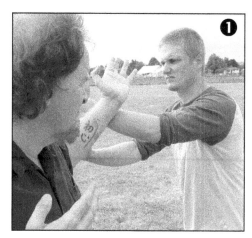

You backhand block the assailant's push or grab.

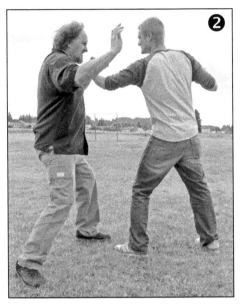

Step out a little if needed and whip a knife hand strike...

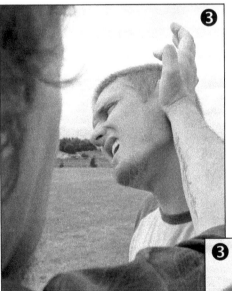

...into his mastoid.

Think through the target.

HAMMER FIST

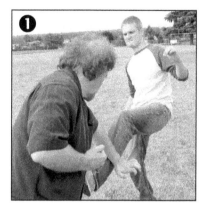

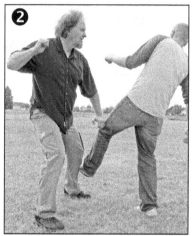

Knock the assailant's kick aside...

...and move slightly to his outside.

Deliver a hammer fist to his mastoid bone. Depending on the height difference, your hammer might travel on a horizontal plain, a downward angle or a slight upward angle.

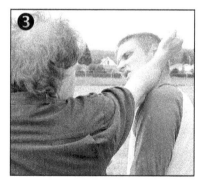

Think through the target.

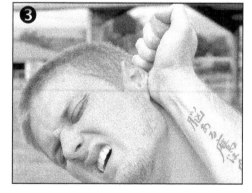

Knee slam

You can deliver extreme force with this technique, thus making the injury potential high. Use it only when you're justified and only after other techniques have failed.

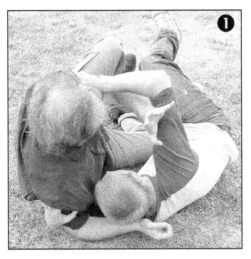

You're fighting on the ground with an attacker who has defeated all your holds and is beginning to overpower you.

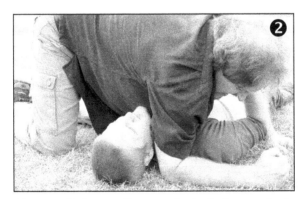

When you find yourself perpendicular to the assailant, quickly stabilize his head with your arm so it doesn't move when you hit it.

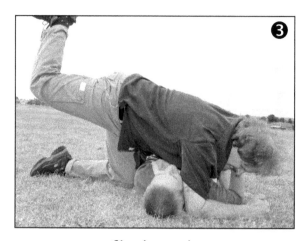

Chamber your knee...

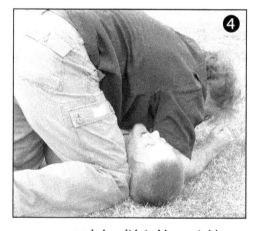

...and slam it into his mastoid.

EARDRUM

A hard blow to the ear shocks the eardrum, causing pain, possible rupture, dizziness and loss of balance. Of course, the impervious person won't feel the pain, or not much, anyway, but he can still be affected by light-headedness and poor equilibrium, enabling you to follow with additional blows or a takedown. If you successfully rupture his eardrum, you will likely take out one of his senses: hearing. If you rupture only one side, you will affect some of his hearing. As long as it discombobulates him, one side is good enough, as every little bit helps.

Potential Injury

A hard blow to the ear can injure the eardrum within, the bones underneath, the bones behind the ear, the inner ear (which houses sensors of position and balance), and the bones and ligaments within the neck. A ruptured eardrum is the most common interior damage and usually heals without treatment within a few weeks or as long as five months. Occasionally, it might require surgical repair to promote healing. Broken bones will also require medical treatment.

The head weighs eight to ten pounds. When the ear is struck forcefully, the neck's job is to stop the head from moving beyond its normal range, a task that can violently stretch and tear ligaments, muscles, and damage nerves.

As always – be justified.

Your objective is to shock the assailant's inner ear so that it confuses, disorients and upsets his balance, at least for a moment, so you can follow with additional blows, a takedown or make your escape.

WMDs

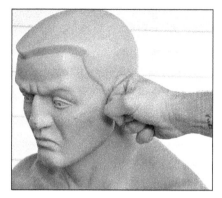

A straight punch to the ear will certainly do the trick but at the risk of injuring your knuckles and wrist.

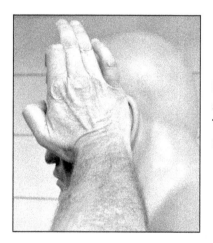

The palm-heel is a safer technique. Notice, that I turn my hand a little to strike with the inner edge of my palm. This reduces the chance of tweaking my wrist.

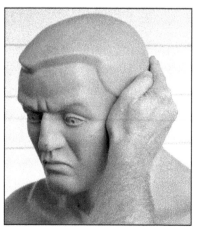

The cupped palm creates a vacuum around the ear that causes immense pain (if they can feel it), possible eardrum damage, and loss of balance.

DOUBLE EAR SLAP

There isn't a women's self-defense class out there that doesn't include this strike. While many techniques taught to women are sadly not the best, this is a good one. The trick is to find that window of opportunity to get the weapon to the target.

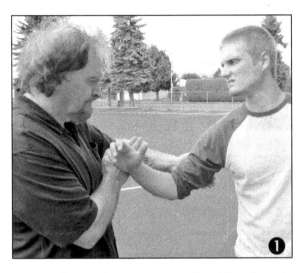

The assailant grabs at your chest. Check it and reach for his upper arm.

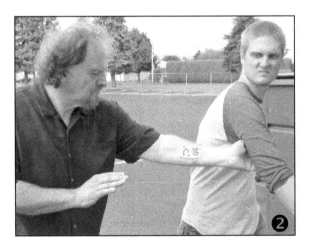

Grab it with a thumbless grip (should he jerk away, there is less chance of injury to your thumb when all five fingers are together), and yank him around...

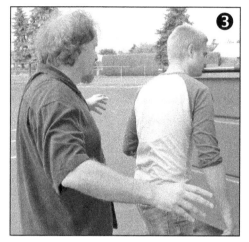

...as you simultaneously step behind him. Double slap his ears...

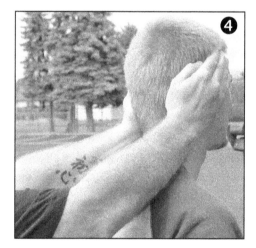

...with cupped palms.

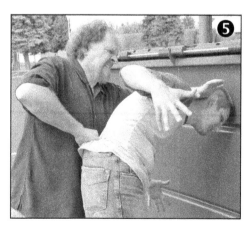

Take advantage of his dazed brain and ram him into the Dumpster.

TACKLE INTO A WALL

The assailant drives you into a wall as he tries to tackle you.

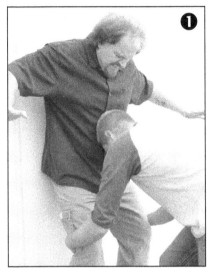

The wall helps to keep you balanced and upright so that you can...

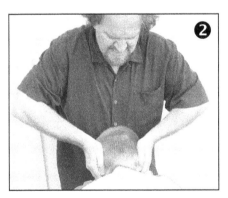

...double slap his ears with cupped hands.

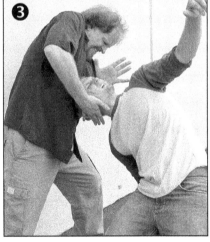

Now that he's dazed and confused, turn his head like a steering wheel and take him down. Flee.

Ear Slam on the Ground

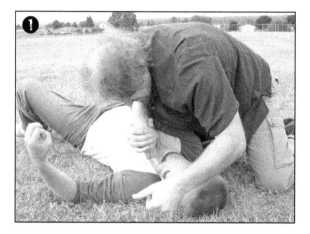

You're thrashing around with the assailant...

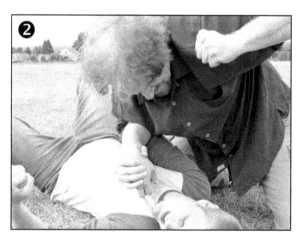

...when that window of opportunity opens. Bang his ear with your:

Options:

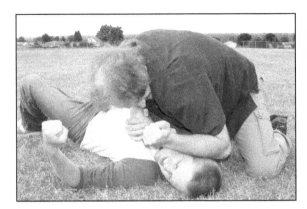

Option 1:
Forearm...

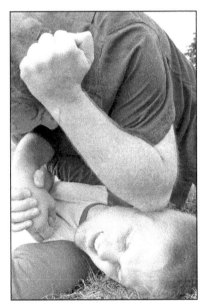

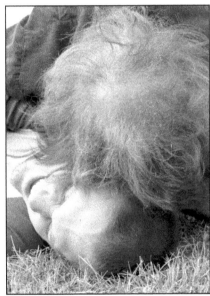

Option 2: Elbow.

Option 3: Forehead. Hit with that part of your forehead that would be covered by a headband.

CHAPTER 3
EYES AND NOSE

If the assailant can't see he isn't worth a darn in a fight. I've said this before in books and it's still true. Three-month-old babies poke their adoring coochie cooing parents in the eyeballs all the time. White belts can do a Three Stooges version after only one lesson.

An eye poke, flick, scrape or gouge will garner some kind of a reaction, even in those people who are pain resistant (this is why doctors check for a corneal reflex before pronouncing a patient dead). While it's hard to imagine that someone can tolerate such a technique, they're out there among us. Thankfully, they're rare. However, while these oddballs might not scream and sob like the rest of us when we catch a finger in the eye during training, they will nonetheless react with tearing, excessive blinking, and/or partial loss of vision. This is precisely the result you want out of the technique so that you can follow up with blows or flee.

The Legal System

Because your average juror has nothing in common with Rambo, she is likely to squirm in her seat and cluck her tongue with abhorrence as you rationalize from the witness stand why you stuck your fingers into someone's eyes. This is because the juror can more easily identify with the agony of a poked eye than the reality that someone can be impervious to pain. It's important, therefore, to not only be justified to use this technique but to know how to articulate why you did. Be able to explain that:

- your pain-based techniques didn't stop him.
- he was continuing to assault you.
- at that precise moment, his eyes were the only target available that you thought would get a reaction.
- your intent was not to cause permanent damage but to distract him so you could flee or take him down.

KEY CONCEPT

Note: Because I have written extensively about the internal conflict within most of us about attacking another person's eyes, I won't write about it again here. The interested reader might want to check out my DVD *Vital Targets: A Street-Savvy Guide to Targeting the Eyes, Ears, Nose, and Throat* for a good discussion on the issue, and a demonstration of a couple of training exercises I learned from an U.S. Army Special Forces officer that help overcome this psychological hesitation.

Let's look at a few eye techniques that force most pain-resistant attackers to blink, flinch and tear up.

ARMS-FREE BEAR HUG

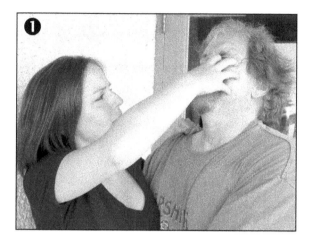

When an assailant fails to react to your head blows and his powerful grip on you is unbreakable, immediately switch tactics and rub your fingers back...

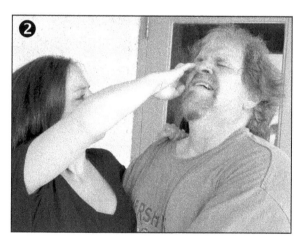

...and forth across his eyes.

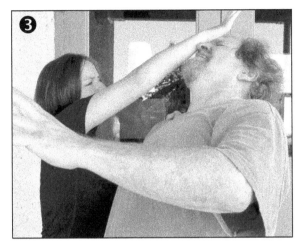

When his grip weakens, push his head back and over...

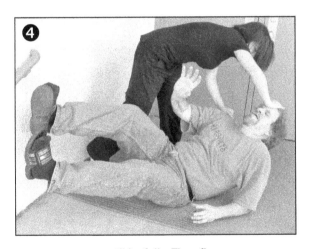

...until he falls. Then flee.

ARMS PINNED BEAR HUG

You had the presence of mind to lift one or both of your arms when he grabbed you in a bear hug.

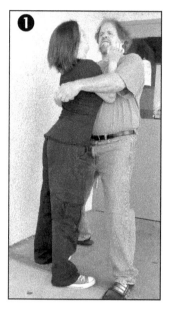

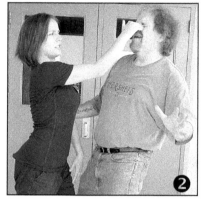

The instant you feel a weakness in one side of his bear hug, ram that hand upward and thrust your fingers into his eyes. Gouge until his grip weakens enough for you to get away.

Your hand or hands are close to the attacker's face.

BEAR HUG FROM BEHIND

He's holding you with one or both of your arms free. You probably have only one chance at his eyes before he pulls his head back and out of the way.

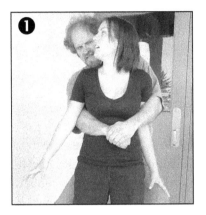

Quick peek over your shoulder to see where his head is. If it's not there, it's probably behind your other one.

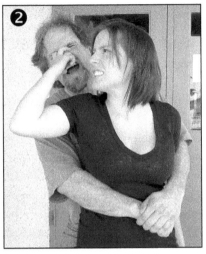

Thrust your hand over your shoulder and into his eyes.

Break free of his weakened grip and flee.

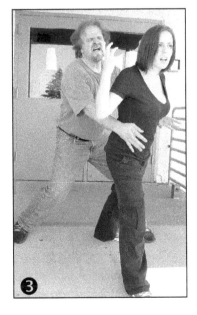

TAP OR FLICK

The problem with an obnoxious and intoxicated person latching onto you - on the street, at a party, in a bar - is that the distance between just being annoying and being violent can be a short trip for a drunk. Here is how it can happen.

"Hey, hey, hey," the drunk says, latching onto a wad of your shirt at a party. "Lishen. Lishen, you! I don't shinkk joo really know whatch happenin' in this country. The democratz are...what was I...I forgets what I'm sayin'."

You try to pull away, but he tightens his grip as he gestures more and more wildly with his free hand. When you try to wrench his arm away, he tightens it so hard that you can't move. You try to squeeze the tip of one of his fisted fingers but he doesn't react to what should be intense pain. When his flailing arm nearly knocks over a lamp, it angers him so much that he begins to yank you about. Is he about to hit you? Should you wait for him to throw a haymaker and hope your defenses work? Or should you act now before it's too late? If you choose the latter, consider a simple eye tap or flick, which are designed to startle the aggressor or, at the least, make his eyes tear up enough to distract him and allow your escape.

Note: The purpose of these techniques is not to injure, but to distract.

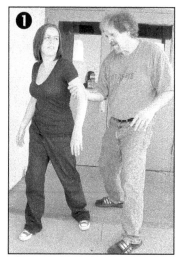 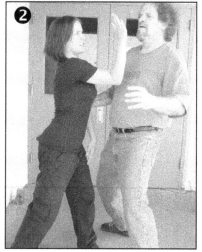

1. A stupid drunk has latched onto you and ignores your verbal requests to let go. He tightens his grip when you try to break free. 2. Flick your fingers...

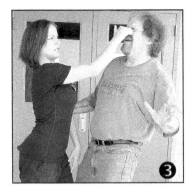

...into his eyes. When his distraction weakens his grip, pull your arm away.

If you don't want to touch his eyes, tapping the corner of one might startle him enough that he releases his grip. However, if he is "out of it," the startle message probably won't reach his pickled brain.

Options:

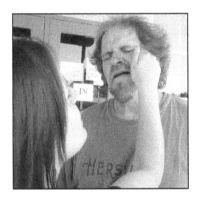

Option 1 (left): Tap with all four fingers at the corner of his eye.

Option 2 (below): Flick a finger (as if flicking a crumb off your lap) against the corner of his eye.

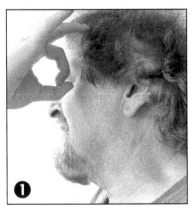

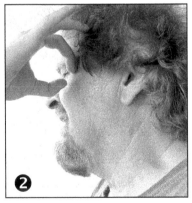

DEFENSE AGAINST A FIST BOMBARDMENT

In sport fighting arts – MMA, boxing, muay Thai – there are lots of good drills where the puncher pummels away at the defender who shields his face and body with his gloved fists. Sometimes this is done as an aerobic drill: The puncher goes nuts on his desperately covering training partner until the hitter runs out of steam and the defender can no longer lift his arms. This is good training – for the ring.

While the shield block is applicable in the street, it isn't for long. Why? Because it hurts! You might be able to take a couple of bare knuckle hits on your arms (if the blows don't numb your limbs and make you drop your guard), but the odds are slim that you can absorb a barrage and then fight back with debilitated limbs.

To state the obvious, a person bent on hitting your face wants to hurt you. If that person is in a drug- or alcohol-fueled zone as he pummels away madly against your forearm shield, you need to counter in a way that penetrates his mindset, and you need to do so quickly to save your arms, and the rest of you. An attack to the eyes will at the very least give him pause and you an opportunity.

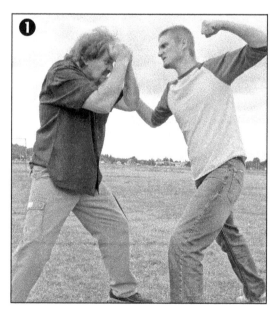

An attacker grabs you and begins wailing on your shielding arms.

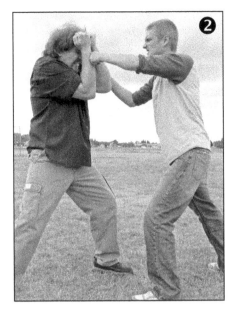

First, give quick thanks that he's stupidly tied up one of his weapons, then lunge forward, using your shielding arms as a penetrating ram to get in...

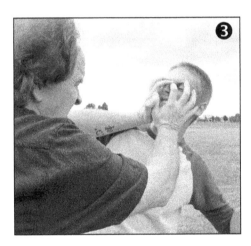

...to claw his eyes...

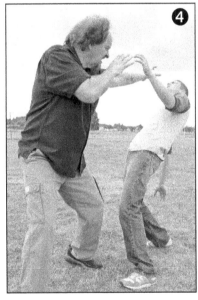

... and force him back. Then flee.

HEADLOCK ON THE GROUND

Because you're not engaging in sport here or thrashing around on a soft mat, you want to end this quickly before his technique turns into a sleeper.

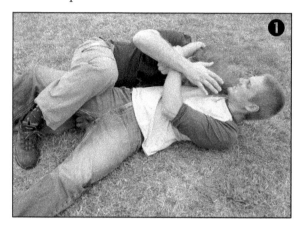

The attacker has you in a tight headlock.

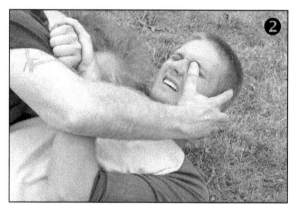

When you have a pathway, ram your thumb into his eye and...

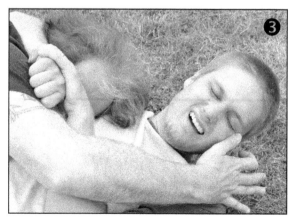

...rip your thumb out to the side. Repeat if necessary. Flee.

ASSAILANT ON TOP STRUGGLE

This isn't sport. You must end this quickly.

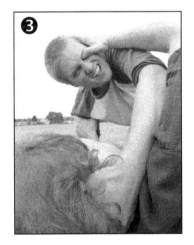

The attacker has taken you to the ground and the two of you are struggling for dominance.

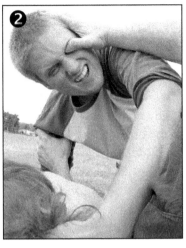

Ram your thumb into his eye and...

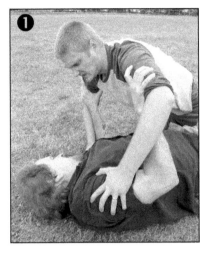

...press with vigor as you...

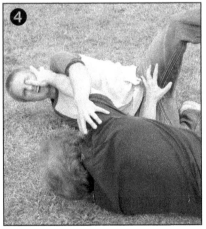

...simultaneously buck him off.

GRAPPLING EXERCISE

As you practice your grappling, be mindful of all the opportunities that occur in your training when you could slip a finger(s) into your opponent's eyes had the situation been real, and he was impervious to pain or greatly superior to you in strength or skill.

NOSE

By now, most everyone knows that you can't drive the nose up into the brain. However, a hard punch or kick there can knock it over to one side, damage the nasal septum (the division between the two nostrils inside the nose), and injure the cartilage, nerves and mucous lining.

If you haven't experienced a hard hit to the nose it's hard to grasp how much misery it brings. Try this: Tap your nose with your fist. Come on, do it harder. Hurts a little, doesn't it? Now imagine a big, outlaw biker's boot kicking it. Incredibly, there are people out there who can tolerate hard hits to the nose and keep right on fighting. We see this all the time in full-contact competition. After a match, an interviewer will comment on the poor man's nose, on how it's lying flat against his left eyebrow. The oblivious fighter, who hasn't looked into a mirror yet, will reach up, feel around and, mutter, "Dang, you're right. I need a latte."

Not acknowledging a shot to the nose in the ring is most often a result of the fighter's raging adrenaline. Five hours later when the shattered-nosed fighter comes down from his high and that horrific pain comes-a-visiting, he begins thinking about getting a nice peaceful job, like selling flowers on the street corner.

A street assailant might not notice your nose shot because he too is on an adrenaline high, a drug or alcohol high, or in a violent, pain-tolerant mental state. (You know it's your turn in the barrel when your assailant is experiencing all of these things at once.) That's the bad news. The good news is that no matter what the reason for someone's inability to feel pain, a blow to the nose will usually make him flinch, blink rapidly, or tear up, at least for a second or two. That is your window of opportunity.

A Brief Open Window

When an assailant is thinking about himself, he isn't thinking about you. Say you're facing someone who does feel pain. He woofs that he's going to this and that to you, to which you nod and smile. Then you bop his nose. Everything suddenly changes for the guy. He's no longer thinking about doing things to you; now he's thinking about the agony in the center of his face. That's when you dump him.

But a pain-tolerant mind doesn't focus on the struck nose. The attacker will flinch a little or a lot, and then his eyes will fill with tears. The blow might not redirect his focus off of you but it might create a distracting physical effect: bleeding, difficulty breathing and vision-debilitating tears. That is your open window to attack.

Note: Your assailant might experience all of these things, just one of them or, though rare, none of them. Expect anything. Follow up immediately when the window opens.

KEY CONCEPT

STRIKE AND KNEE CATCH

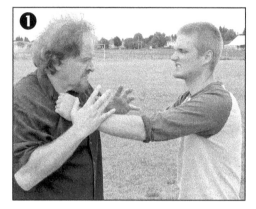

The instant the attacker grabs a wad of your shirt, react by...

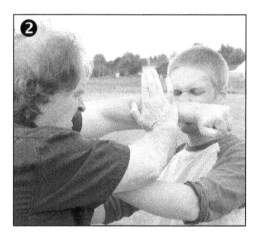

...slamming your supported forearm into his nose. Twist your hips and drive with your rear leg for maximum power.

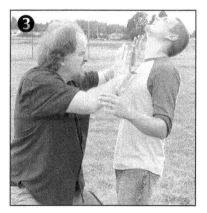

Though he doesn't feel the pain, take advantage of his one- or two-second reaction by...

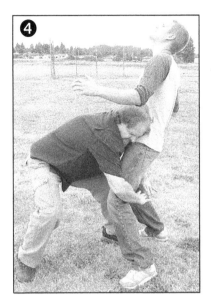

...dropping to catch his knees. Pull them toward you as your ram his middle with your shoulder.

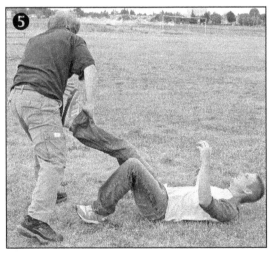

Down he goes. Flee.

SPIN, THUMP, RUB

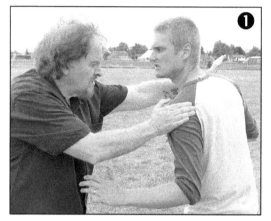

To disorient him, spin him about by pushing one shoulder and pulling the other.

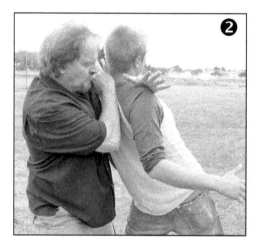

In this case, the left pushes and the right pulls. In the event he doesn't spin as much as you want, step behind him as he turns. Your pulling hand moves up to create a brace behind his head...

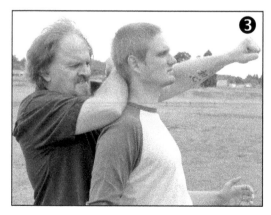

...as you extend your other arm.

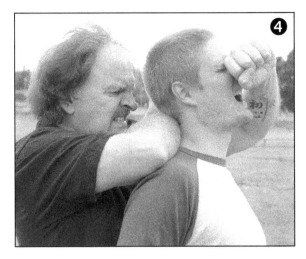

Then retract it hard and fast to impact his nose.

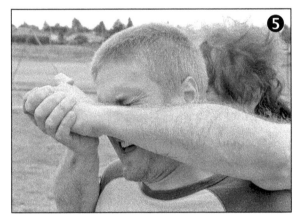

Clasp hands and saw your forearm back and forth. In this case, begin at your wrist and saw it...

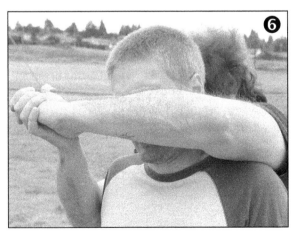

...five or six inches toward the middle of your forearm, then back. Saw as many times as you can to encourage eye watering and to activate numbed pain sensors. Then throw him to the ground.

THUMP, RUB AND THUMP AGAIN

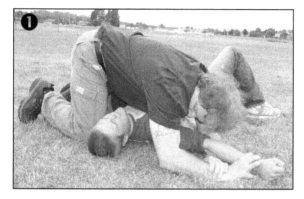

He doesn't feel your armlock, or you're applying it incorrectly, and he begins to bend his arm.

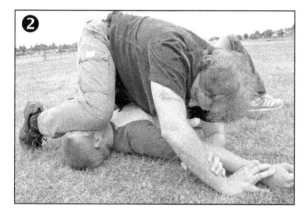

Quickly drop your shin onto his nose...

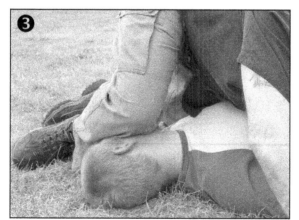

...and rip it across his face. His head will turn in the direction of the rip.

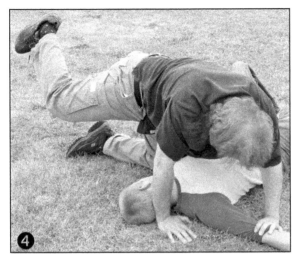

Brace his head and chamber your knee.

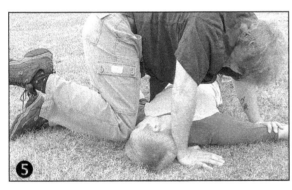

Slam it into his nose. Your objective here is to make it difficult for him to breathe and to "blind" him with heavy tearing. Get up quickly and flee.

CHAPTER 4

BRACHIAL PLEXUS, VAGUS NERVE,

THROAT & BACK OF THE NECK

Be justified to strike an attacker anywhere on the neck. Consider this incident.

A 24-year-old casino security guard attempted to stop a man from betting with other people's winnings. A fight ensued and the guard managed to throw the man out of the establishment. An hour later, the unruly patron returned and commenced to throw punches at the guard, which he blocked. The guard then delivered a single punch to the man's neck, sending him to the floor, unconscious. The man was whisked away to the hospital where he was pronounced dead on arrival. The security guard was promptly arrested and taken to jail.

The outcome of the guard's arrest was unknown as this book went to press.

BRACHIAL PLEXUS

The brachial plexus stun is an incredibly effective technique on most people who do feel pain. While you probably won't get the same results hitting a person who doesn't feel anything, it will still debilitate him to some degree.

THE BLOW MUST BE ACCURATE

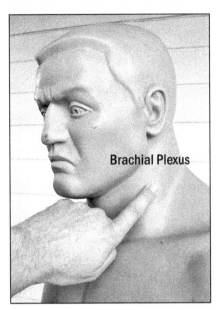

Brachial Plexus

The brachial plexus is located on both sides of the neck half way between the front and side. If the attacker can feel pain, hitting him in front of or behind the exact point will hurt, but it won't have the same debilitating effect as hitting directly into the nerve cluster. A poorly aimed blow on a pain-resistant person might not slow him at all.

Warning:
A Blow to the Throat
can be Fatal.

Why mention the throat in a discussion about the brachial plexus? Because unless you're immobilizing the attacker's head as you fire in a blow to the side of his neck, he can easily turn at the last moment and inadvertently expose his highly fragile throat. Might you then be held answerable for his serious injury or death? Yes. This is why it's critical that you're justified to use this technique, or any technique.

CAUTION

USE A HEAVY, PENETRATING BLOW

Your blow should land heavily so that it penetrates deeply before it retracts. In contrast, a snapping blow hits the target and is pulled back immediately, delivering—and this is arguable—less energy.

Your blow should stay on target for about ¾ of a second—longer isn't better—to allow the fluid shock to penetrate the nerve cluster and generate its nasty effect. I find that hitting the brachial plexus with the inner or outer forearm works nicely.

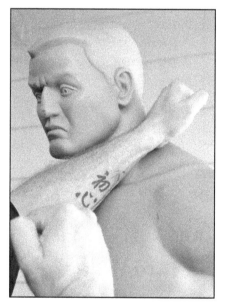 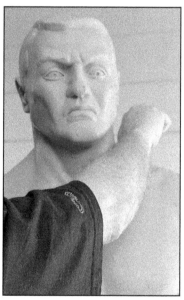

Outer forearm strike.   Inner forearm strike.

When coupled with a drop step, the arm hits fast, hard and stays on target for nearly a second. You can also hit with a backfist, hammer fist, knife hand, foot or shin.

Snapping blows, such as a snapping backfist, are generally considered a less effective way to hit the brachial plexus. That said, a friend snapped a poorly controlled backfist to his training partner's neck and sent the hapless fellow to his knees where he tried to remember if it was Christmas or the 4th of July. Although there are always exceptions, the ¾ of a second policy seems to be most effective.

My friend, Officer Steve Holley, a veteran cop who counts the brachial stun as one of his favorite techniques, told me of an incident that he witnessed. A 240-pound bouncer, who stood well over six feet tall, was working in a tough bar in a southern state when a group of pro football players walked in one day, dwarfing him with their steroid-fed gorilla physiques.

Of course steroids, beer and group psychology make for a bad mix, and soon the bouncer was confronted by one of the giant football players just outside the door. When the drunk raised his hand threateningly, the bouncer slammed the inside of his right forearm into the man's left brachial plexus, sending him to the floor with a loud *plomp* and a raised cloud of dust.

The bouncer then stepped over the downed man, pointed at the next closest players, and asked, "You want some of this?" They wisely backed away.

When the big football player went down, the back of his head hit the floor so hard it could be heard by Officer Holley inside his police car as he rolled up to the scene. Fire department paramedics couldn't get the man to respond, so he was flown to the hospital by a medical helicopter where he was diagnosed with a concussion.

THE EFFECTS OF THE BLOW

I once asked a student to hit my right brachial plexus so that I could get a sense of what it felt like. Using a scale of 1 to 10, 10 being the hardest impact, I asked him to hit me with a blow between a 1 and a 2 (it's not that I'm a coward, I just don't like pain). I backed up to a chair and waited for him to drop his forearm against the side of my neck.

His blow ignited a brilliant flash of light in my head similar to a camera flash, followed by an awful throb of pain streaking through my neck, head and shoulder. I fell back onto the chair, and tried to reach toward the agony, but my right arm ignored the commands from my brain. My neck hurt, my arm was at once numb and hurting, and my entire right side felt "funny," but not the ha-ha kind. My student, laughing the entire time, said that my eyes were spinning like reels in a slot machine.

The moment lasted about 20 seconds, a period in which I couldn't have responded defensively if my student had continued attacking. After 20 seconds I was able to move about and probably could have defended myself. However, I was left with a horrendous headache that lasted for nearly an hour.

I've been hit in the brachial plexus in training, though not quite as hard as my student whacked me, and although it gave me pause, I was able to keep going. On the street, a pause by your assailant is a good thing.

Martial artist and physician, Dr. Matt Hing, explains that although the area contains five nerve roots, a heavily intoxicated drunk man might not feel a blow there.

"These are peripheral nerves and alcohol intoxication dulls the central nervous system, making everything numb for the drunk. When he wakes up from his stupor, though, he is in for a lot of rude pain from brachial plexopathy (torn nerves) if, in fact, the plexus was torn from the impact. On the other hand, if you do sufficient damage to the brachial plexus, you might so disable the person's ability to control the muscles in that arm to the extent that you are now fighting an essentially one-armed opponent. In other words, your blow will stun the arm, but not the crazy man."

There is likely to be some mental confusion, too. It can be considerably disorienting and even distracting for the opponent to realize that his body is not responding to commands from his mind, especially since he can't relate this inability to pain. To him, his brain has stopped functioning, at least the way it had been before you hit his neck. Might this make him more violent? Maybe. Or it might make him more flustered, which can work to your benefit.

Keep in mind that there are no absolutes when dealing with the human body. Anyone who says that if you hit here or kick there that there *will* be specific results is sadly misinformed. Throw out all absolutes and expect anything.

Let's look at some ways to hit the brachial plexus.

OUTSIDE FOREARM

The argument against blocking with two arms is that by committing two weapons to block, you might not be able to defend against a follow-up hit. This is a good point if you're slow. But if you have good hand speed, you can block, strike the brachial plexus and be back on-guard within a second. Never is this more important than when you're blocking inside as is the case in this scenario.

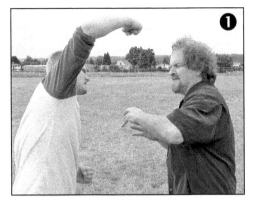

The attacker throws a sloppy right.

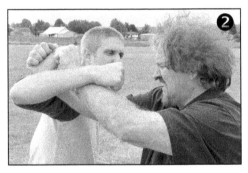

Block with both arms and then...

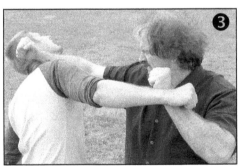

...explode off his arm into his...

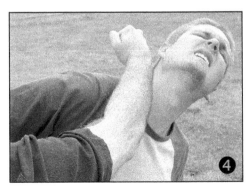

...brachial plexus with the outer edge of your forearm. Flee.

INSIDE FOREARM

You can generate tremendous whipping action with the inside forearm strike. As always, be justified.

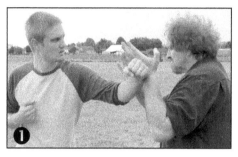

You're in a mirror stance when he throws a left jab. Block it with both hands.

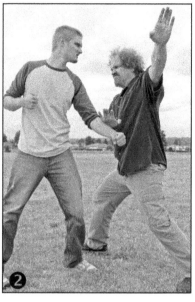

Jam his arm out of the way as you begin to drop step with your right foot and prepare to strike with your left forearm.

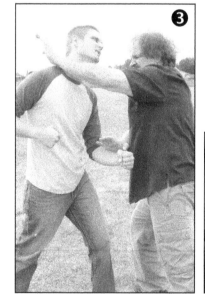

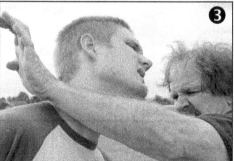

Your foot should land heavily as you slam the inside of your forearm into his right brachial plexus.

Point of impact.

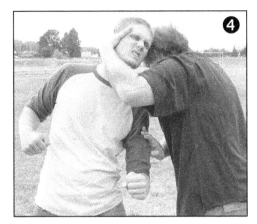

If needed, cup the right side of his face and...

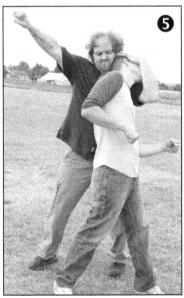

...pull his head to the side. Chamber and...

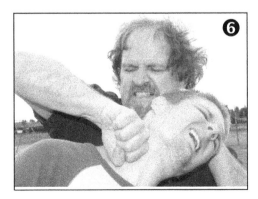

...slam a right thumb-side fist into his exposed brachial plexus. Then flee.

Here are two scenarios in which the assailant tackles at different levels. Each one requires a different defense weapon.

Low TACKLE

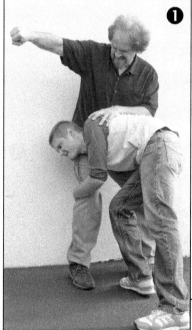

The assailant comes in low and drives you into a wall. Slam your forearm...

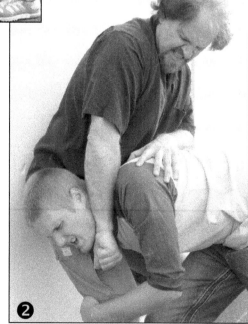

...into his brachial plexus. Since it's hard for you to see the exact target from this position, you might have to strike repeatedly until you hit it.

TORSO TACKLE

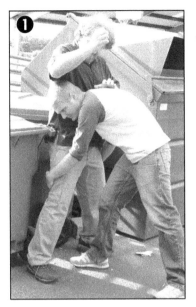

The assailant tackles you and drives you into a Dumpster.

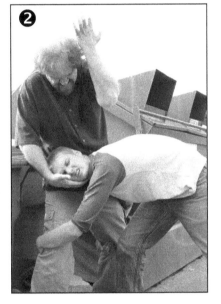

Crank his head to the side to disorient him, create a base for your hit, and expose his brachial plexus.

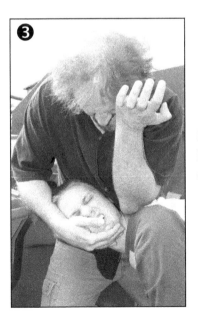

Ram the point of your elbow into his brachial plexus. Push him to the ground and flee when he weakens.

In the preceding "Inside forearm," you saw one way to get behind an attacker to hit the brachial plexus. You can also use any of the body twist methods shown previously or, if he is threatening or attacking a third party, you can approach him from behind. Here is a way to do it when defending against a kick.

FOREARM STRIKE FROM BEHIND: BLOCK AND SPIN

Block/sweep his kick with enough force to turn him.

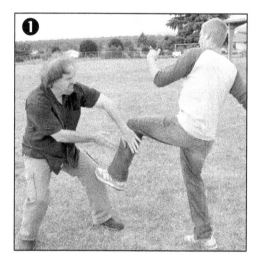

He kicks at you. Sweep his leg aside and....

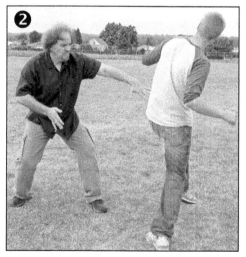

...move behind him.

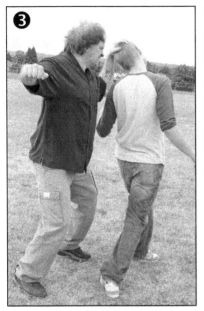

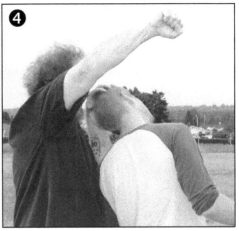

...and slam the inside of your forearm

Pull his head down to expose his brachial plexus...

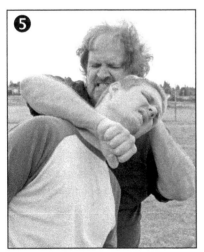

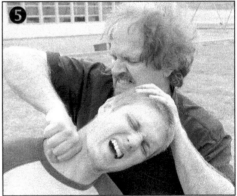

Option: You can also hit him with the thumb side of your fist.

...into the target.

KICK TO BRACHIAL PLEXUS

There is great potential to cause serious injury when kicking someone in the neck. Be justified. Be justified. Be justified.

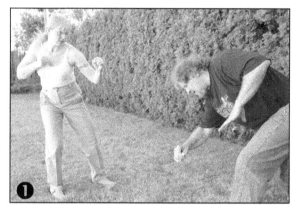

The intoxicated attacker swings his knife, loses his balance...

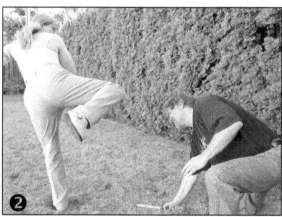

...and drops to one knee. This is your opportunity to flee. If you can't run, seize another opportunity to attack. Kicking a knife-wielding attacker is always a risk since he can move his knife faster than you can kick. But if he is 1) heavily intoxicated, 2) you possess exceptionally fast kicks, and 3) the attacker's weight is on his weapon arm as pictured, whip a...

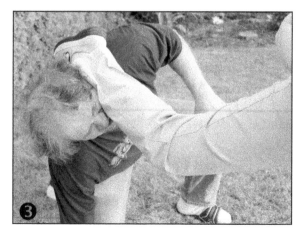

downward-angled round kick (hit with your shin) into his brachial plexus.

When fighting on the ground, you have less mobility and fewer options to escape. If the attacker is more skilled than you at ground fighting, he's impervious to pain, or he's superior to you in strength, a strike to his brachial plexus might reward you with a few seconds to follow-up or get up.

THE ATTACKER IS IN YOUR MOUNT (LONG RANGE)

Take advantage of any moment in which you have one arm free, or both, and a clear path to the target. You will be able to do this when you have trained to respond instantly to a brief window of opportunity. Conversely, if you haven't drilled on it, you probably won't respond in time, or you might not even recognize the moment.

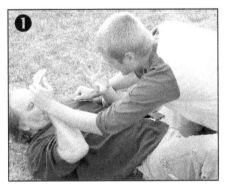

You're hand fighting for dominance.

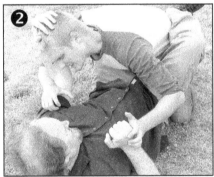

Suddenly, your left is free. Grab the side of his head to brace the target and...

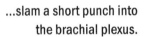

...slam a short punch into the brachial plexus.

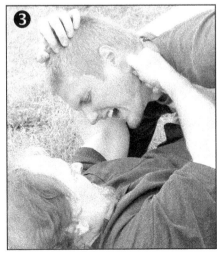

THE ATTACKER IS IN YOUR MOUNT (SHORT RANGE)

In this similar situation, you pull the attacker's head into you or he lowers it against your chest by his own accord. Your other hand is being restrained and can't brace his head. Your blow will still work, though it might require two or more hits.

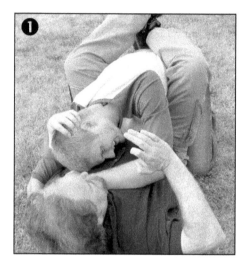

The attacker lowers his head into your chest. Strike his brachial plexus using the best weapon for the job.

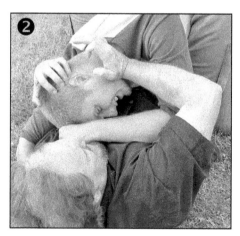

In this case, a knife hand thrust easily slices into the small space.

YOU'RE IN THE ATTACKER'S MOUNT

You're in a good position to inflict damage, but he isn't feeling it and he's starting to get the best of you.

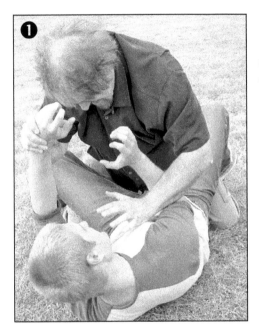

As you battle for dominance...

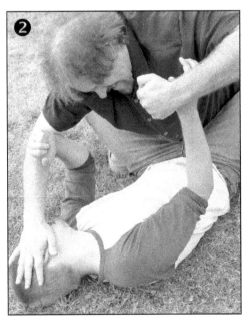

...seize the moment to press his head to the side to expose his brachial plexus. Choose the best weapon for the angle and range. You can:

Options:

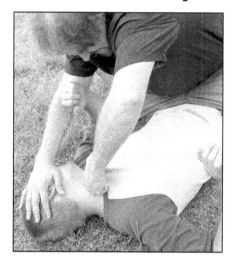

Option 1: Hit with your fist.

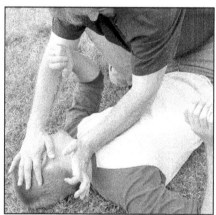

Option 2: Hit with the edge of your hand.

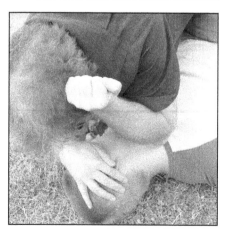

Option 3: Hit with your elbow.

SIDE STRUGGLE: FORCE HIS HEAD INTO POSITION

You and the attacker are on your sides struggling for dominance. You see an opportunity to force his head into a place where it can be hit.

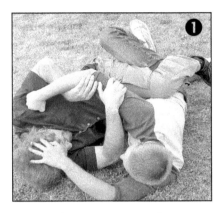

The two of you are wrestling for control.

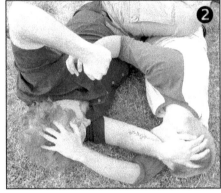

When the moment is right, push or pull his head to expose his brachial plexus.

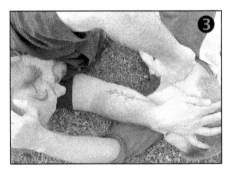

Strike it with the best weapon given the distance and position, such as punch...

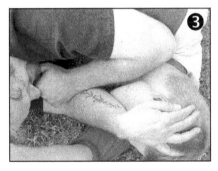

...or an elbow.

Side struggle: Take advantage of his position

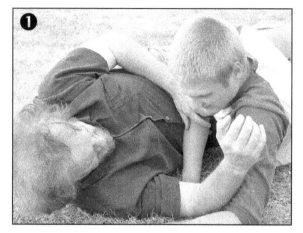

During your struggle, he lifts his head just right to expose his vulnerable neck.

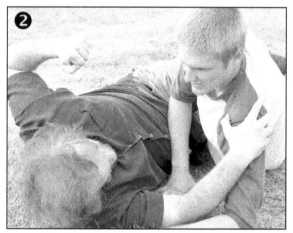

Seize the opportunity...

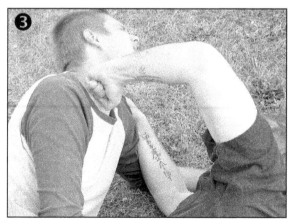

...to hit his brachial plexus with the best weapon.

VAGUS NERVE

Latin for "wandering," the vagus nerve emerges at the back of the skull and wanders all the way to your abdomen. Before it gets there, it does some branching out along the way, making contact with your heart, lungs, voice box, stomach, ears, and a few other parts. It wanders by the brachial plexus and the carotid artery, so it's hard to hit one without hitting the others, and that's okay. As the saying goes: "It's all good."

When the vagus nerve is stimulated via massage, your heart rate slows and sometimes your breathing. When it's stimulated by a hard blow to the neck, there can occur what is called a "vaso-vagal response," meaning that the recipient's heart rate and blood pressure drops so low that he feels feint, he actually feints, or he slips into a coma. He could also die. Be justified.

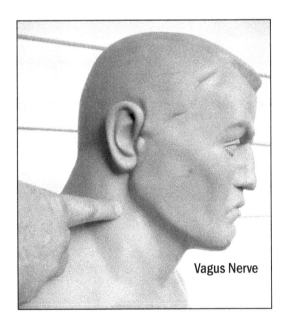

Vagus Nerve

BEAR HUG

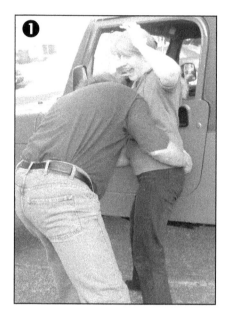

The assailant grabs you in a sloppy bear hug...

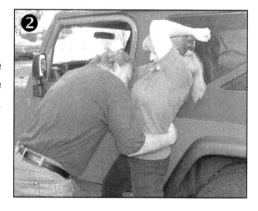

...and slams you against the side of a car. Take advantage of your free arm...

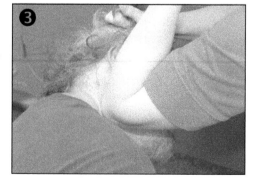

...and spear the point of your elbow into his vagus nerve.

INSIDE CAR

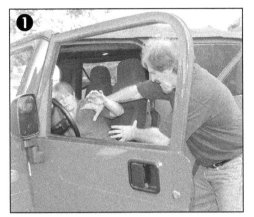

A drunk follows you out of a restaurant and jerks open your car door.

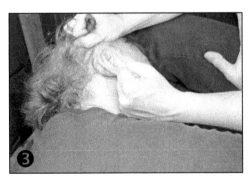

Block his grab and pull his head downward to pull him off balance.

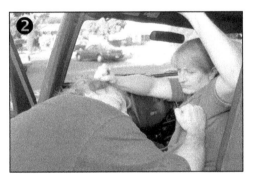

Strike his vagus nerve once (in this case with a hammer strike).

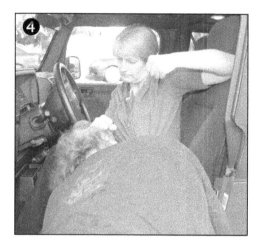

Should you want to hit it again, and your position changes a little...

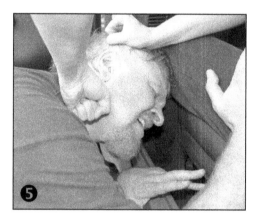

...hit him with a different strike (a fist in this case).

Note: Any technique used to hit the vagus nerve will work to hit the brachial plexus.

THROAT

Both of the men were drunk and combative. I was not feeling well, so weak that it was difficult to lift my arms, let alone fight back against the most aggressive one who had grabbed the front of my shirt. The guy had already driven me back against a large plate glass window that bowed inward from our combined weight, and I was fearful that it might break if he shoved me again. So I punched him in the throat, a quick and short right hand that dropped him to his knees instantaneously, and sent his frightened buddy running off into the night. Although, the drunk could feel pain (judging by how he was carrying on), I punched the dangerous target because I had no gas to fight, I didn't want to be sliced open by that window, and I knew a throat punch would drop him.

A blow to the front the throat can damage the thyroid, Adams's apple, even crush the trachea (windpipe), cricoid cartilage, or damage the laryngenial nerves that could lead to suffocation. I'm guessing that I hit my assailant with about 25 percent of my power, if that. More would have likely injured him severely or even killed him.

Be justified to hit this target.

When you strike a pain resistant assailant in the throat, the very least he will do is gasp for air and choke. That is your window of opportunity to follow-up with blows to other targets that weaken him, or to execute a takedown technique.

THROAT SLAP

A slap has less penetrating power than a punch and, therefore, might be less injurious while still causing the assailant to cough and gasp.

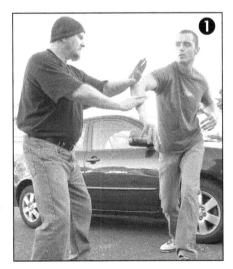

You block his punch.

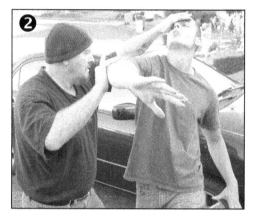

Lunge step beside him and slap your palm against his forehead.

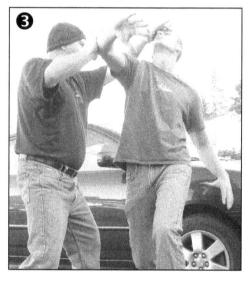

Push his face and arm upward to disorient him, and then force him...

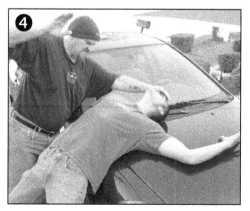

...down to the ground or onto a car. Chamber...

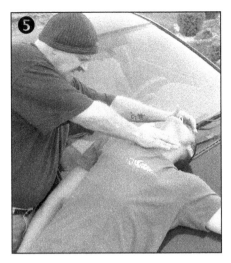

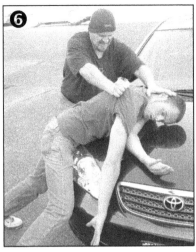

...and slap. It's not necessary to hit with full force.

When he begins to wheeze, push him off...

...the car and flee.

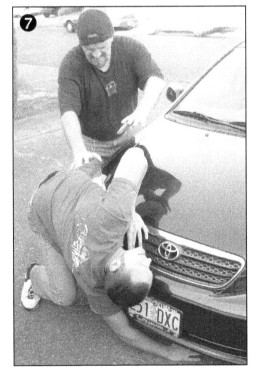

SLAP FROM BEHIND

You're behind the assailant on the ground. Seize the window of opportunity.

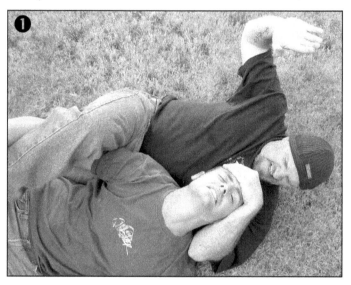

Pull his head back. Before he can resist...

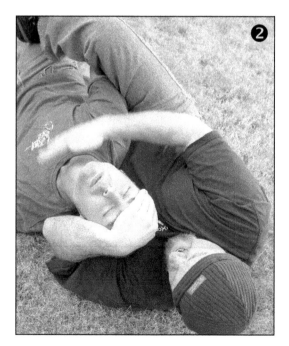

..slap your palm...

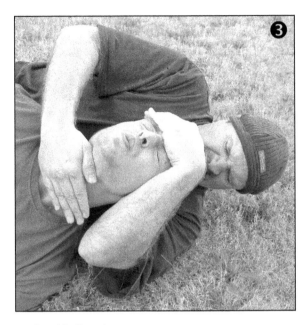

against his throat.

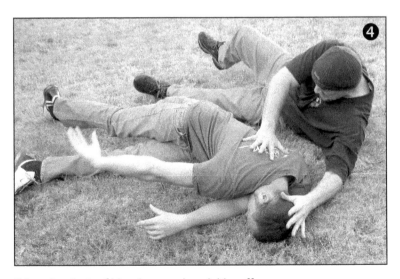

Take advantage of his misery and push him off you.

FINGER-BONE STRIKE

This is sometimes called "tiger's mouth," and other names, but it's nothing more than striking with the outside bone of your index finger. The web between your thumb and index finger catches some of the impact but mostly the bone does the hitting.

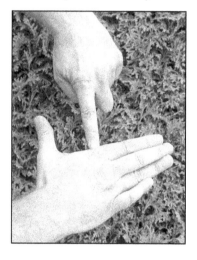

Index finger bone. Hit with a quick out and back snap.

Let's say you have gone to the ground several times with the assailant and everything you have tried has failed to have an effect.

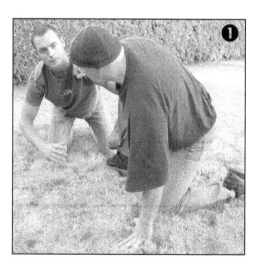

You're both on the ground and you're trying to make an escape. He follows and grabs your pant leg.

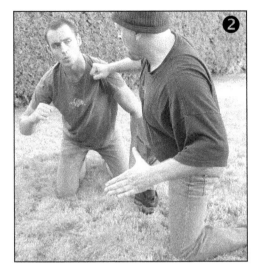

The angle of his head and neck are perfect to...

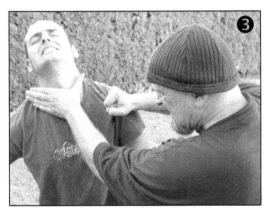

...hit with your finger bone.

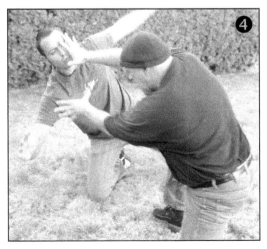

Then push him down.

BACK OF THE NECK

A powerful blow to the back of an assailant's neck can cause mental confusion, paralysis, breakage, or death. In most cases, your objective is to affect only mental confusion so that you can flee or dump him. The problem is that it's hard to know what the affect will be. Hit one assailant's neck and he staggers about in confusion. Hit a second assailant and his neck breaks. Although it's the assailant who created the situation in which you're forced to defend yourself, you will still be held responsible for the outcome of your blow. Be justified.

TIGHT BEAR HUG

Sometimes this is called a "ghost hit" because the recipient doesn't see it coming. Earlier, we looked at striking the external occipital protuberance, the bony ridge on the lower skull, but above the neck. Both are good targets.

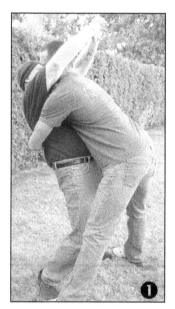

The mentally deranged assailant embraces you in an arms-free bear hug and begins taking you over backwards to the ground. Immediately extend your arms and clasp your hands.

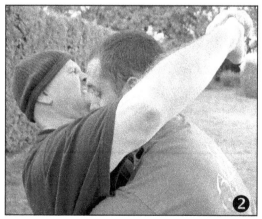

As you fall, use your left hand to help slam your right forearm...

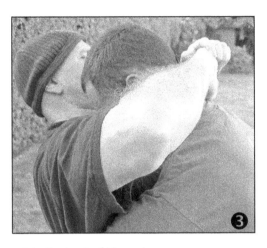

...into the back of his neck.

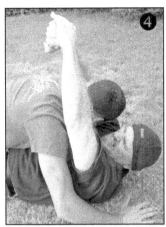

If necessary, hit him again...

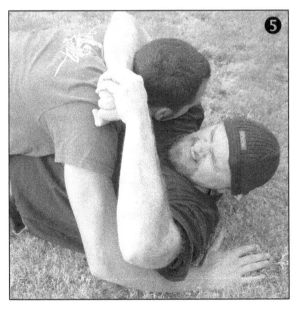

...after you're on the ground. Then push him away and flee.

CHAPTER 5

CAROTID ARTERY CONSTRICTION

The common carotid artery supplies the head and neck with oxygenated blood. The arteries begin at the heart and travel upward along each side of the neck. When constricted, the blood supply to the brain is slowed, not stopped as is often believed. You can affect a sleeper hold by constricting one or both arteries. When it's applied just right, the recipient will lose consciousness within seconds.

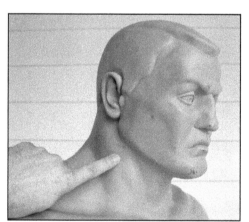

Constriction is placed at this point on one or both sides of the neck.

Consider these stages.

- You will feel the attacker's body become slack and then go completely limp.
- Immediately relax the constriction but *do not give up the hold* until you're able to flee or you have help to restrain him.
- He might be out for only five seconds, or 30. He might be faking it.
- Some people awaken passive and confused, while others come around still fighting.
- Maintain the hold *without constricting his arteries* until you can determine his demeanor. Should he wake up fighting, you're in position to constrict again.
- When he goes out the second time, again release the constriction but not the hold.

Note: Continuing to constrict the attacker after he loses consciousness might cause brain damage or death. *If he doesn't awaken from your constriction, immediately call for an ambulance.*

APPROACH FROM BEHIND

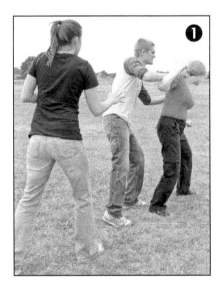 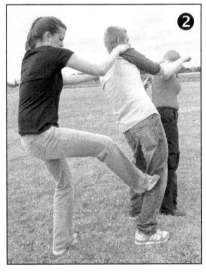

You approach a violent person who is attacking your friend.

To take him off balance and to lower him a little, slam your foot into the bend of his knee as you yank his shoulders back and down.

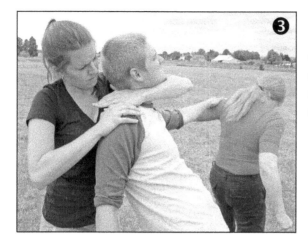

Slip your arm around his neck keeping your elbow elevated.

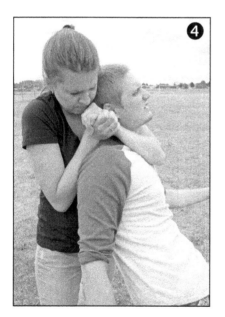

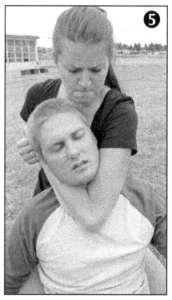

Clasp hands and slam your forearm onto his chest to drive him down.

Your upper arm constricts one artery while cartilage on the inside of your wrist constricts the other. Push with your hand to tighten the constriction.

Option:

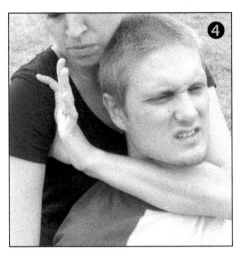

Insert your thumb into your armpit and...

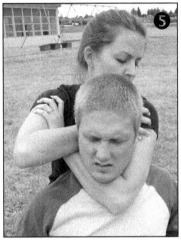

...extend your other arm across the back of his head. Grab your other shoulder or, if you can't, make the effort to reach for it (this tightens the constriction).

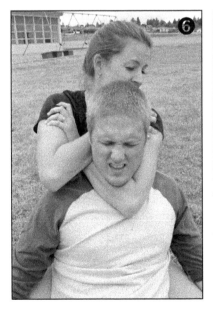

Squeeze both elbows toward each other to constrict his arteries.

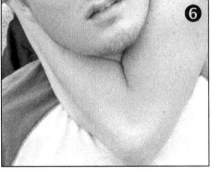

The elbow of your constricting arm is centered under the attacker's chin so that pressure is applied to both arteries, rather than against the front of his throat.

GROUND

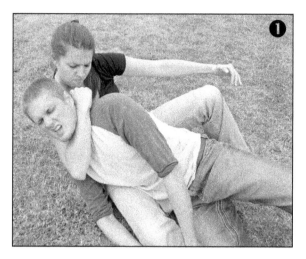

You're thrashing around on the ground with an attacker when you find yourself behind him. Seize the opportunity to encircle his neck...

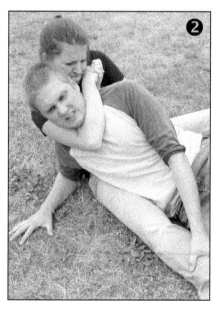

...and apply the constriction.

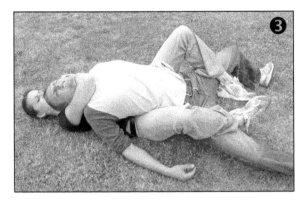

Either hook your heels inside his legs to control his lower body or... ...

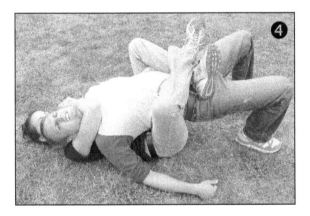

... scissor your legs around his lower waist. Flee when he becomes groggy or completely loses consciousness.

TRAPPED ARM SLEEPER

This is a tight constriction, though its weakness is the somewhat awkward wrist grab. Practice until you can do it smoothly and then look at other ways to get into it.

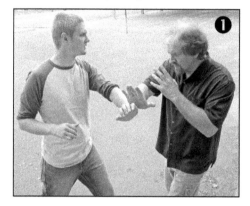

Palm aside the assailant's reaching arm, but maintain contact with it.

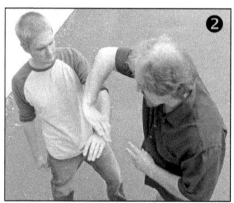

This is the awkward part - at first. Rotate your hand so that you're gripping his hand with your four fingers on the little finger side of his hand.

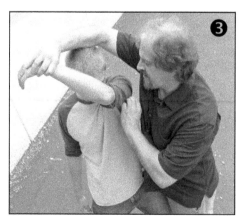

Loop your arm over his head so that his hand and arm are at the other side of his neck.

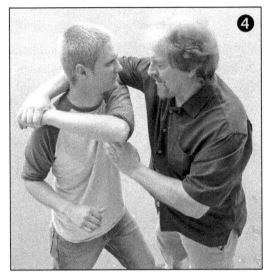

Slip your other hand...

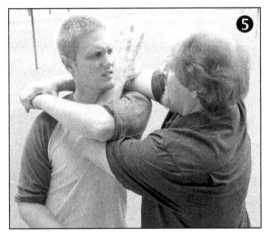

...between his face and your arm.

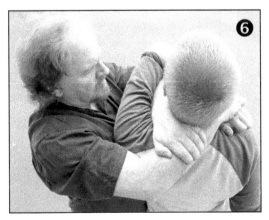

Clasp your forearm.

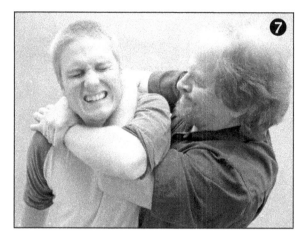

Both of your wrists are now positioned against his carotid arteries. To constrict them, pull his wrist toward his opposite shoulder.

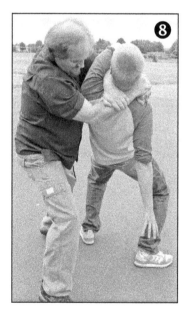

When he goes limp...

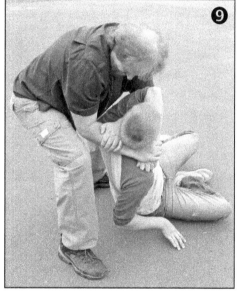

...lower him to the ground gently. Dropping him could injure his head.

CHAPTER 6
HEAD AND NECK COMBINATIONS

While most of us fantasize about delivering that one-punch knockout, the reality is that such a thing is quite rare. The solo knockout blow is often, perhaps most often, the result of a lot of factors coming together at the same time:

- Power
- Speed
- Distancing
- Precise position of the target
- Precise position of the impact weapon
- Vulnerability of the target
- Momentum behind the blow
- Movement of the target into the impact
- And other elements

Since it's difficult to deliberately arrange for all these things to occur at the same time, it's best to combine blows. This is especially critical when dealing with an atypical opponent, one whose pain sensors have been turned off.

It's easy to get into the mindset of thinking that any target is a good target. While this is somewhat true when the adversary is capable of receiving messages from all his pain receptors, it isn't true when his cloaked brain is blocking incoming pain signals. In fact, it can be risky to hit just any target because it might waste precious time and leave you open for a counterattack.

Let's look at a few simple combinations against some of the specific targets that have been discussed in this section.

Double ear slap

To brag for a moment, I've got a powerful slap (a result of a lot of cross-body cable work), so that makes this one of my favorites. Not only are you double impacting the assailant's eardrums, but you're forcing his brain to bounce around inside his skull. While he might not feel the pain, the double blows will likely discombobulate his thinking and disturb his balance.

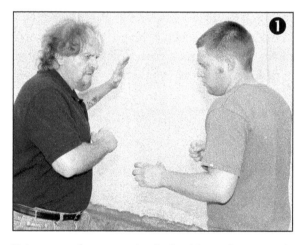

Using power from your chest, shoulder and arms, and power generated by the rotation of your hips...

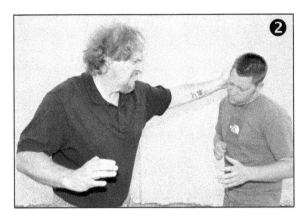

...slap your cupped hand against an attacker's ear.

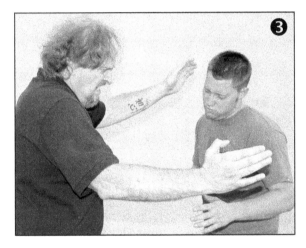

Just as his head and brain are moved as far as they can go...

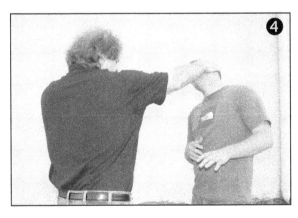

...slam your other cupped palm against his other ear. If there is an opportunity and a need, strike the first ear again. Take him down and flee.

HEAD BUTT, HAMMER FIST

React quickly when bear hugged to avoid being pinned by a powerful person who can tolerate pain.

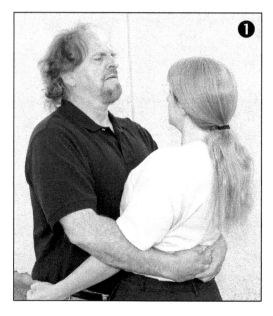

The attacker grabs you in an arms-pinned bear hug.

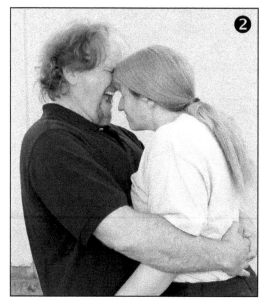

Headbutt his nose and then...

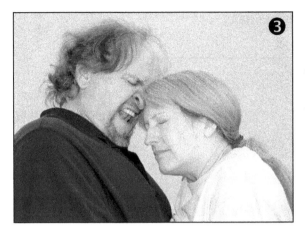

...grind your forehead into the injury to underscore the tearing effect.

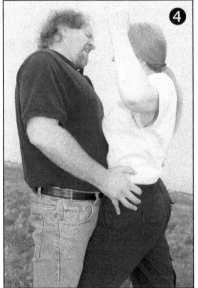

When he leans away, take advantage of his weakened grip to...

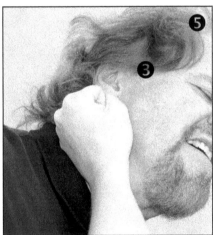

...slam a hammer fist into his brachial plexus. Flee.

STRIKE THE BACK OF HIS HEAD

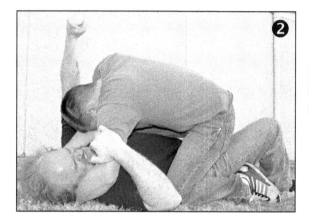

The assailant is on top and dominating you.

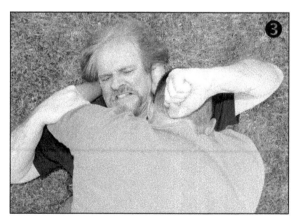

Extend whichever hand is free over his head.

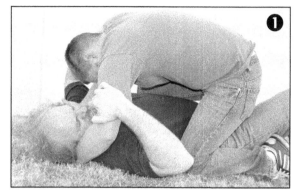

Slam the thumb-side of your fist hard into his external occipital protuberance, that bony ridge just above his neck. Repeat if needed.

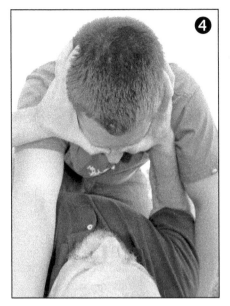

Then thumb his eyes...

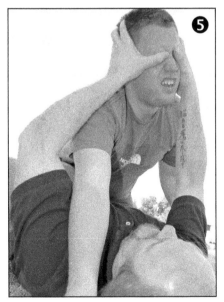

...to force his head back.

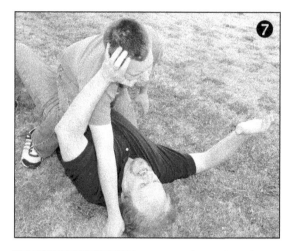

Support one side of his head...

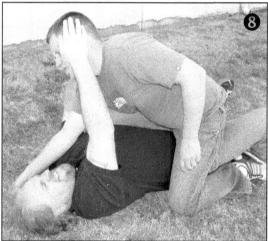

...and slap your cupped hand against his opposite ear.

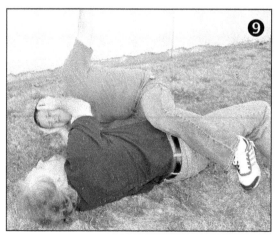

Buck him off into the soil.

A WINDOW OPENS

Windows of opportunity are short lived. When one opens…
move!

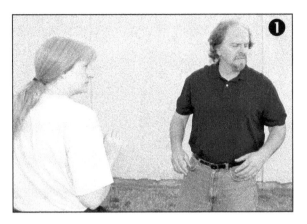

The assailant is distracted by something off to his side. Then he blinks.

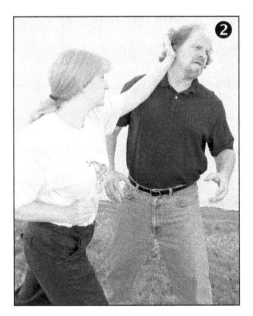

As quick as his blink, ram the edge of your palm into his mastoid, that…

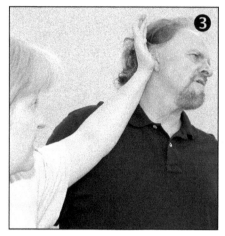

...bony ridge behind his ear.

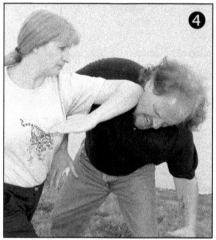

Continue moving forward as you fold your arm into an elbow strike against the side of his neck in the area of his carotid artery, vagus nerve and brachial plexus.

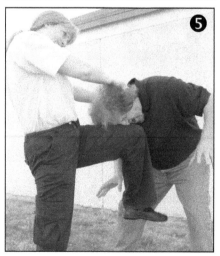

When his dazed head drops, pull it into your knee strike. Flee.

THREE DOUBLE-HAND STRIKES

The window of opportunity opens for three double hits to debilitating targets.

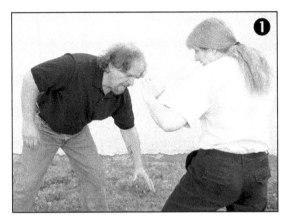

The attacker loses his balance for a moment. That's your window.

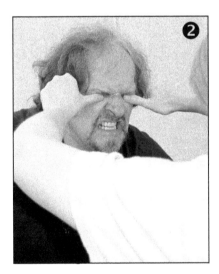

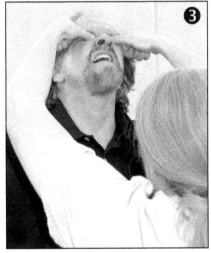

Lunge forward with a two-handed finger gouge to his eyes.

Push his head up.

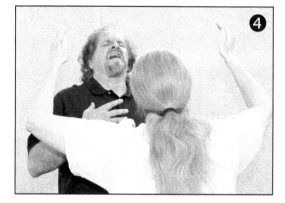

Quickly chamber your hands...

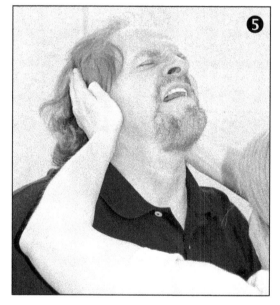

...and slam double-cupped palms against his ears.

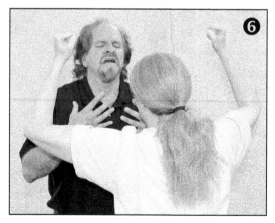

Chamber again as he staggers...

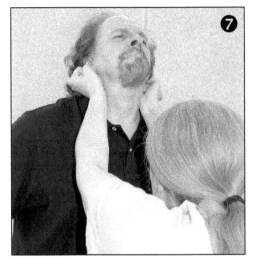

...and double strike his brachial plexuses.

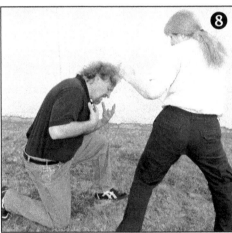

Back away and flee as he withers to the ground.

Note: This is the only place in which I combine a few techniques from the material just discussed. I encourage you to put together combinations of torso and arm targets, leg targets, and throws. Then once you're comfortable with those, combine techniques from all the chapters. Your objective is threefold:

- to train to develop seamless delivery of techniques to high, low and medium-high targets.
- to execute takedowns.
- to understand the medical implications of the various targets.

CHAPTER 7
TORSO

There are good targets on the torso that when struck will cause debilitation, though the attacker might not feel pain. The problem is that people cover these targets with heavy coats several months out of the year. The only time people cover their faces is when they're on an expedition in Antarctica or robbing a 7-11. So when the assailant is wearing a heavy coat, refer to the head, neck, legs, and takedown chapters. When he is dressed in a T-shirt, a Hawaiian shirt, or he is shirtless like one of those mentally deficient subjects on the *Cops* TV program, consider the many torso shots noted here.

THE SOMATIC REFLEX ARC

This is a nifty human phenomenon that begs for you to exploit. Although I've used it for years, I didn't know it had a name until my friend Steve Holley enlightened me and related how he has used it in police work for years.

For our purposes, the somatic reflex arc is the body's involuntary response to a blow. Gouge a man's eyes, and he snaps his head back and jerks his hands up to protect his face. Punch someone in the kidneys and they arch their back in the direction of whichever one was struck.

This reflex action, which occurs even when the receiver doesn't feel pain, is good news for you because it opens a window of opportunity. When the attacker automatically snaps his hands up to protect his just-poked eyes, he leaves everything from his chin to his toes open for you to do whatever enters your mind. When he arches his back reflexively in response to your kick slamming into his kidney, he is momentarily off balance and ripe for you to take him down.

Let's examine a few of these targets.

SOLAR PLEXUS

Perhaps you have seen fighters knocked out in boxing and MMA from a single punch to the solar plexus. It's always surprising when it happens, although it shouldn't be considering the physiology. The solar plexus (also called the celiac plexus) is a complex network of nerves located behind the stomach directly below the pecs. A hard, deeply penetrating blow there can cause agonizing pain to those who can feel it, it can stop visceral functioning (certain body functions) and—what you want—a sudden forward bend at the attacker's waist.

Will everyone react this way? No. While a soft, fat person usually reacts to a hard solar plexus punch by bending forward, a fat person with a large, hard stomach might not.

KICK TO SOLAR PLEXUS

The attacker moves toward you.

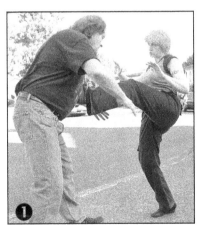

Drive a hard front kick...

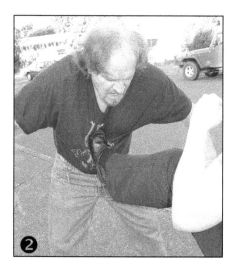

... into his solar plexus

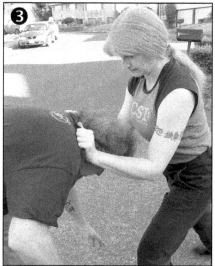

Drop your foot in front and grab his forward-thrusting head, hair or collar.

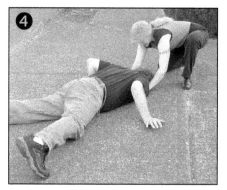

Step back as your drive him down to the sidewalk.

PUNCH TO SOLAR PLEXUS

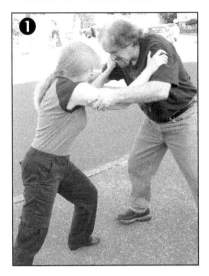

You're scuffling about in a sloppy clinch.

When a pathway clears...

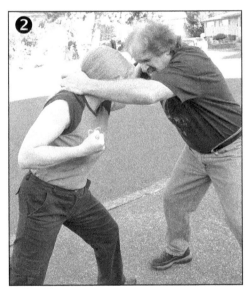

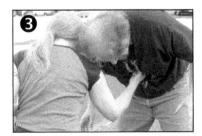

...drive a deep, penetrating punch into his solar plexus.

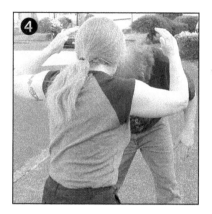

When he reflexively bends forward...

...double slap his ears...

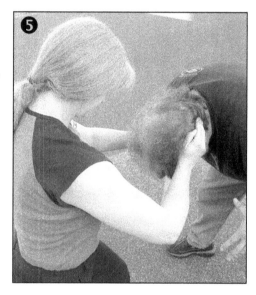

...and pull him down by whatever you can grab.

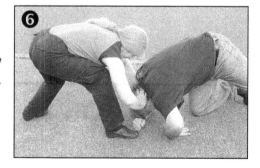

KIDNEYS

If you've been training for a while, you've probably been hit in the kidneys. This can cause horrific pain that some people liken to getting kicked in the groin. One time I got kicked in the kidneys by a dentist. No, he wasn't working on my teeth at the time; we were sparring one another in an all-black belt class. The dentist was a tough fighter with an especially powerful roundhouse kick. My kidneys definitely hurt, but what caused me the most grief was urinating blood and chunks of…I don't know what the chunks were, for exactly 31 days. Yes, 31 days! The doc said the kick broke some things off the walls of my kidney. That's how he said it, too: "The kick broke some things off."

While a blow to the kidney hurts like the dickens and can turn going to the bathroom into a scene from a horror movie, the impervious-to-pain crowd won't feel it. They might the next day when they sober up or come down off their high, but that won't do you any good when an attacker is trying to drag you into the back of a van.

Where It Is And What It Does

Shaped like a big bean, the kidneys hang out in the back part of the abdomen on either side of your spine. Rest your hands on your hips and you will locate them about where your thumbs are. You may be able to actually feel the lower part of the right kidney as you inhale, but probably not the left one, since it's about an inch higher. They are approximately four inches long, two inches wide, and one inch thick. The average adult's weighs four to six ounces. Their job is to remove undesirable substances from your blood plasma, such as toxins, acids, and excessive water. They also conserve water.

KEY CONCEPT

While the pain-resistant attacker might not feel the actual blow to his kidney, he will wonder why he's suddenly sucking for air like a beached fish, since most find it difficult to breathe after getting hit there. While he's wondering and sucking, you want to follow with additional techniques or flee the area.

To activate the somatic reflex arc, the blow needs to penetrate deeply into the kidney, as opposed to a punch that snaps in and out. Think of hitting his stomach by way of his back. Hit hard and accurately, and the attacker will reflexively bend backwards. He does this for only a second, so act quickly to take advantage of it.

Hook, hook, slam

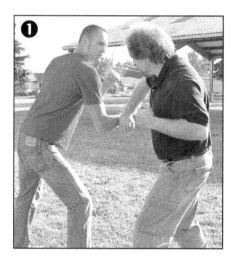 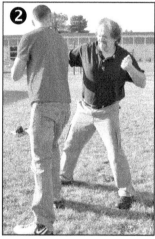

When the attacker tries to push you, hook his arm toward his inside...

...so that it turns him. You might have to step out a little.

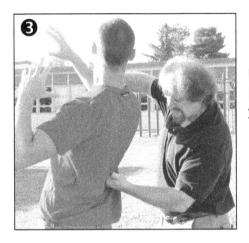

Uppercut or hook punch his kidney once or twice as hard as you can.

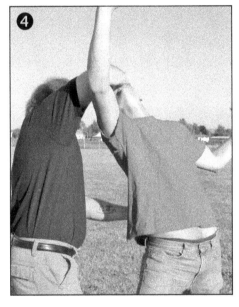

When he arcs back, grab his face...

...and ram him to the ground.

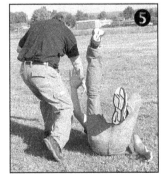

Hook kick, chin push

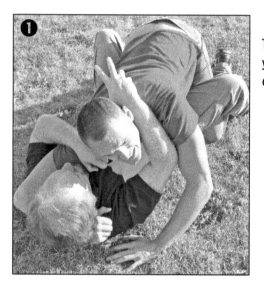

The attacker is on top of you; your efforts to get him off have failed.

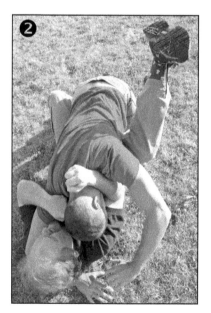

Strike one of his kidneys with multiple heel kicks. (You must possess a powerful hook, a result of lots of repetition training and resistance exercise.)

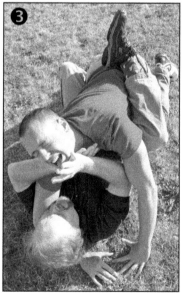

When he arcs his back a little in response, attack his eyes or push his chin.

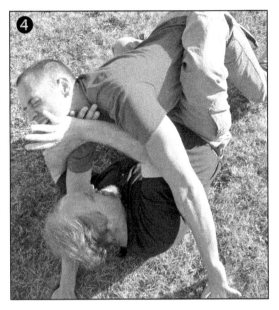

Now that you're in a stronger position, bump him off you.

Scramble away.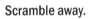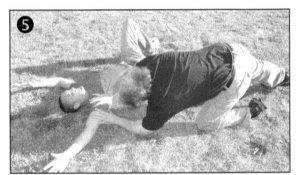

EVADE, HIT, PULL

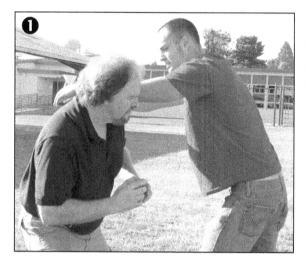

The crazy man reaches for you. Evade to the side...

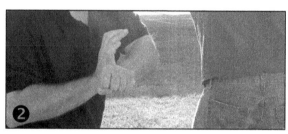

...then move quickly toward his back. Support your forearm with your hand...

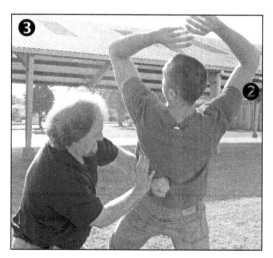

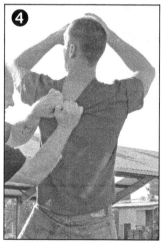

...and drive it deeply into his kidney. Note how his back arches back.

Grab his hair, head or collar, and pull him onto his back. Flee.

LIVER

Full-contact fighters think about punching the liver more often than point fighters because they know the terrible debilitation of a hard punch or kick to this sensitive target. There is nothing quite like the instant nausea, rubber legs and the absolute inability to go on that follows a solid blow to the liver. Typically, a person struck in the liver, even one who is impervious to pain, will pause for a second before he bends backwards or drops to his knees. Sometimes he does both.

The liver is a large organ that lies under and behind your right lung, and extends down to your bottom right rib. It's surrounded by a capsule, which is extremely sensitive to pain caused by trauma. (I saw a book recently where the author an MMA champion, was talking about hitting the liver. His photos, however, depicted punches to the model's left side. To reiterate, the liver is on the right side.)

THE BEST IMPACT POINT

Judging by boxing and MMA fights, the most popular point of impact is that small space just above the right hip bone and just below the bottom rib. Hit too low and you will hit his hip bone. Imagine a line that begins at this point and extends diagonally up to his left shoulder. That is the path of your hit. Your objective is to dig your fist—typically a hook punch—under his rib and drive all the way up to his opposite shoulder.

THE SECOND BEST IMPACT POINT

While hitting below the floating rib appears to be the most popular pathway to impacting the liver, some boxers land their hooks higher up on their opponent's side next to the right pectoral. I asked Dr. Matthew Hing about the two locations, "Both are good targets," he said. "The liver lies deep to the right nipple and extends to just past the lower margin of the rib cage. Hit either location and you jar one of the most vascular organs in the body. The liver is a literal reservoir of tremendous amounts of blood. Of the two sites, hitting under the floating rib is probably more direct and will result in more damage."

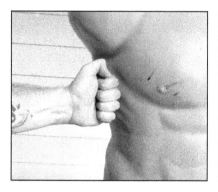

Use a horizontal punch when standing and hitting at pectoral level.

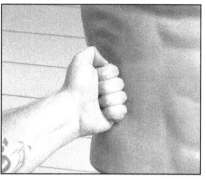

Use an upward diagonal angle when hitting below the ribs.

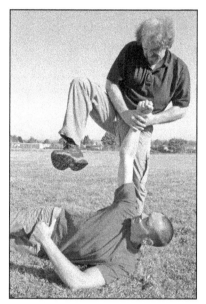

To attack it vertically, punch or stomp straight down...

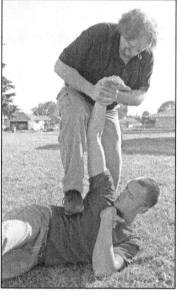

...hitting the ribs anywhere from the pectoral line to just under the bottom floating rib. As mentioned elsewhere, don't straighten your body upward as you stomp down because this moves your energy away from the target. It is better to drop your body weight (and energy) into your stomp.

Here are two ways to hit the lower and more common impact point to the liver.

HIT AND PULL HIM DOWN

You're getting up from the ground as the attacker moves in. Come up swinging.

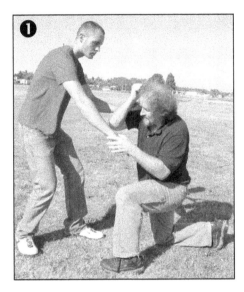

Shield your head with your right arm as you stand.

Lean to the left to load your punch and then drive off your left leg to...

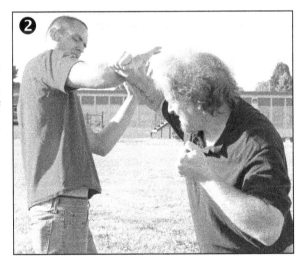

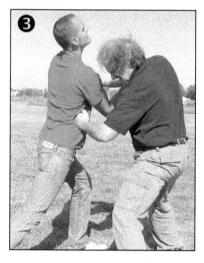

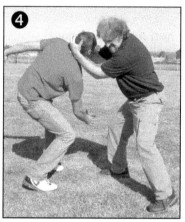

...hit deeply into his liver. When he bends into your hit...

...grab him by his head...

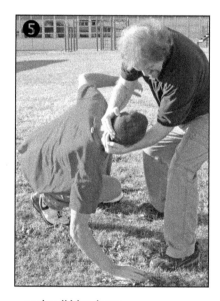

...and pull him down.

Option:

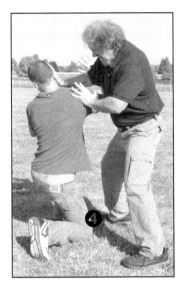

If he drops to his knees...

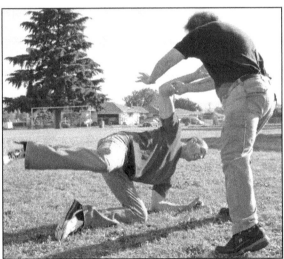

...push him over.

CLOTHING GRAB, LIVER HIT

In full-contact fighting, a good liver puncher might deliberately leave himself open to his opponent's right punch, thus exposing his right side. Since leaving your chin open in a real fight can be risky, consider other opportunities to exploit.

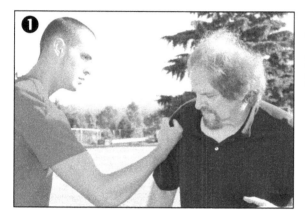

The attacker grabs your sleeve to pull you in.

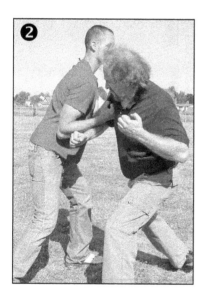

Go with the pull and load onto your left leg...

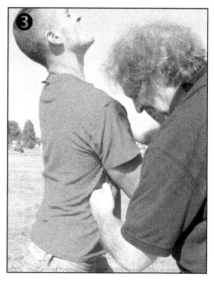

...then shove off of it to drive in a hard hook to his liver.

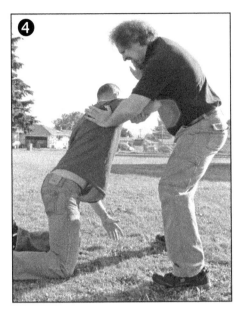

When he drops to his knees...

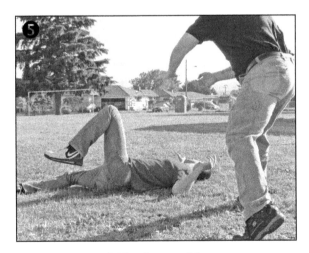

...push him down and flee.

CHAPTER 8
BICEPS, FOREARMS AND FINGERS

When I was in high school, my buddies and I regularly smashed each other in the biceps as we passed in the crowded halls. A hard blow would instantaneously numb the other guy's arm, leaving it hanging from the shoulder like a dead opossum. Sometimes we would hit each other so hard that our biceps would puff up like Arnold Schwarzenegger's in his heyday, all the while they hung uselessly.

The concept here is simple: Take one arm out of the fight and the attacker becomes a one-armed fighter. It's irrelevant that he doesn't feel the pain because the struck limb will die, anyway, for a few seconds to a few minutes, a moment in which you follow with another technique or flee. Cambodian fighting champion Eh Phou Thoung understood this well as he is well-known for kicking his opponent's biceps, sometimes breaking their upper arms.

QUICK SHOT

Sometime all it takes is one powerful blow to activate the arm's delete button.

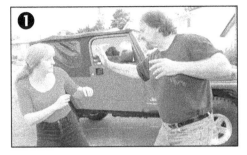

The attacker launches a slap.

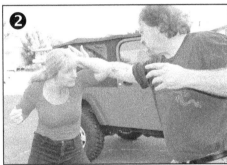

You shield block it and follow...

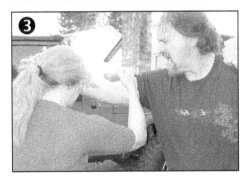

...with a hammer fist to the belly of his biceps. Hit it again if possible.

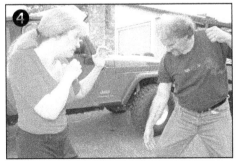

Back away quickly when his arm drops uselessly. Flee.

STOMP HIS BICEPS

You have gone to the ground with the attacker.

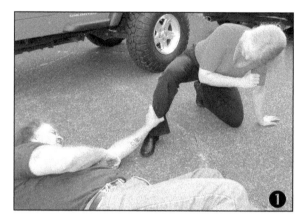

As you scramble to your feet, he grabs your ankle.

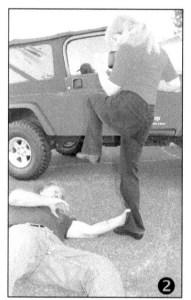

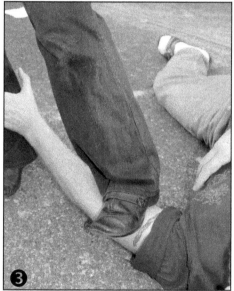

Immediately, stomp...   ...the belly of his biceps, twice if you can.

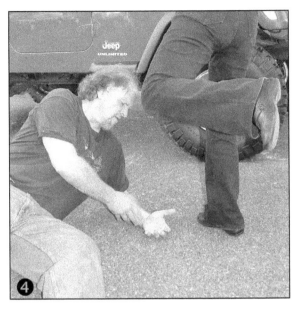

When he leans to that side unable to get up, slam his nose with...

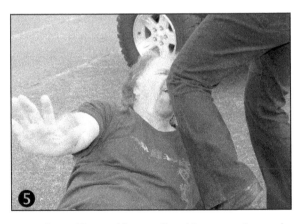

...your knee. Flee as his arm dies, his eyes water, and he struggles to breathe.

HIT BOTH ARMS

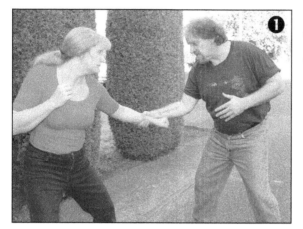

The handsome attacker grabs your left arm.

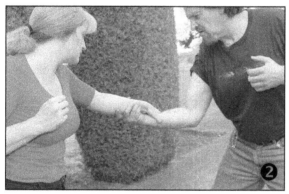

Quickly loop your hand around to brace his arm. (If he is gripping it so tightly that you can't move your hand, that's okay as the rigidity will act as a brace.)

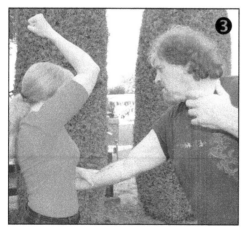

Deliver a powerful elbow strike...

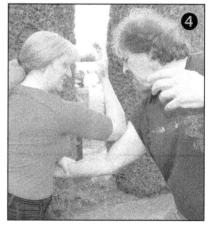

...to his biceps. Again, if you can.

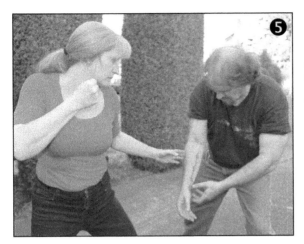

Jerk your arm away from his dying grip and...

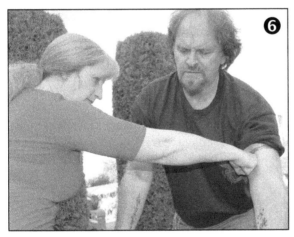

...punch his other biceps...

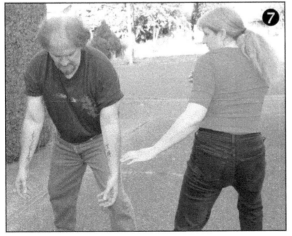

...as you make your escape.

FOREARMS

Have you ever been struck on your forearm, especially the upper portion near your elbow? That's more fun than a human should have, eh? If you were hit hard enough and in the right location, your arm probably felt as if it had been shocked all the way to your finger tips. It might have gone completely numb and dropped uselessly to your side. If you had been holding onto something—an arnis stick, training knife, frappachino—you probably dropped it. This is the reaction you want in a self-defense situation.

I've often used forearm strikes to get resisting drivers to let go of their steering wheels and others to release their grips on weapons, doorframes, and my pant legs. The effect isn't always instantaneous, so hit until you get the desired results. Some might argue that it's not a good technique if you have to hit multiple times. The counter argument is that you're using this technique because it's the best for the moment.

The literature shows that there are multiple susceptible points on the forearm. But to keep things simple, I'm listing only two. As in all the targets we've looked at in this book, the attacker might not feel the pain but he will react to the nerve trauma from your blows. If all is good, his arm will be virtually or completely useless.

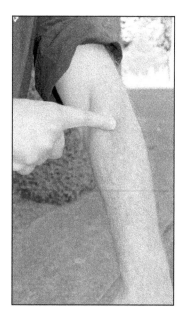

Impact Point 1 is about two inches down the forearm from the elbow crease.

FOREARM STOMP

During the course of the battle, you apply a leverage technique, an armbar.

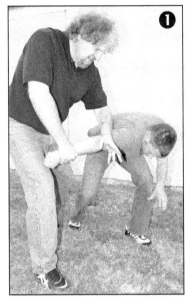

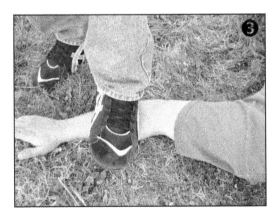

Take him down

The instant the hard landing stuns him, release his arm and chamber your leg.

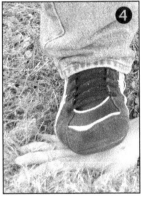

Stomp the beefiest part of his forearm, about two inches below the bend of his arm with the edge of your shoe or its heel. Stomp again if needed.

If you can stomp his fingers, do that, too. The forearm blow will make it hard for him to grip a weapon or make a fist. Stomping his fingers will make it even harder.

Option:

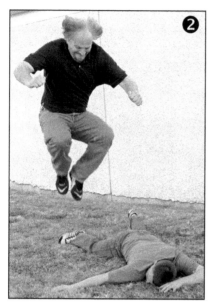 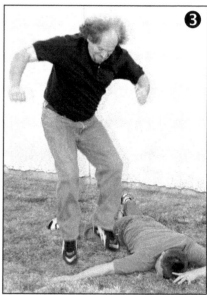

If you got time, jump...   ...onto his...

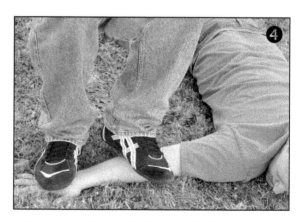

...forearm and fingers. (Grimacing like Bruce Lee is optional.)

FOREARM STRIKE

This works well off a reach or punch. Often, when the offending forearm is struck, the attacker's body will jerk forward. Take advantage of this by following with a forearm strike to the side of his neck. The first strike numbs out his arm, and the second blow to his brachial plexus and vagus nerve numbs out his brain.

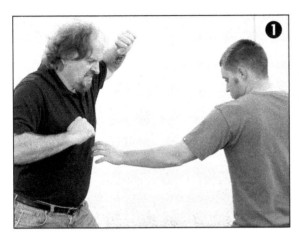

When the attacker reaches for you, chop down...

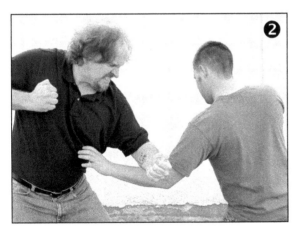

...onto his upper forearm. Think of the impact...

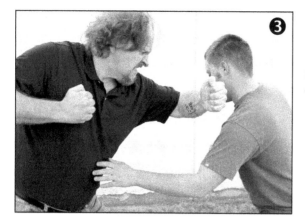

...as a trigger that launches your outer forearm...

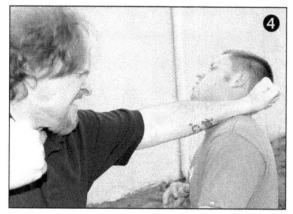

...into the side of his neck.

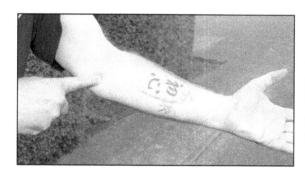

Impact Point 2 can be found by tracing your finger along the crease of your arm until you find the hard protrusion.

Note: If you have a choice, strike the aforementioned Impact Point 1 rather than Impact Point 2. A blow to Impact Point 1 quickly deadens the arm and reduces the attacker's gripping power. Impact Point 2, however, is a little less reliable.

Since this target is part soft tissue and part bone, hit it with your palm to prevent injury to your knuckles.

TAKEDOWN ASSIST

You're applying a takedown technique that relies on leverage as opposed to pain. You also want to take his arm out of the equation.

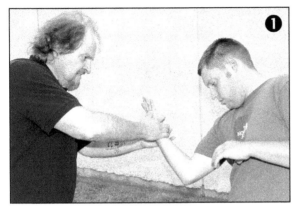

Grab the attacker's hand and twist it...

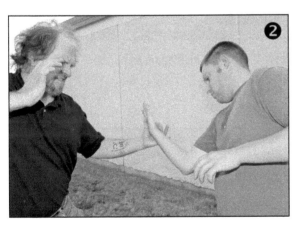

...for a takedown. Take advantage of the exposed forearm point...

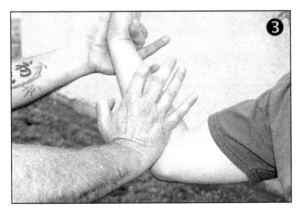

...and palm-heel...

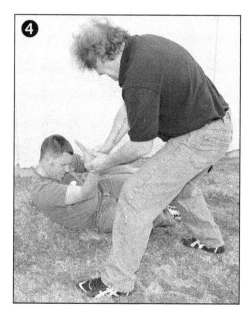

...strike it. If possible, hit it again as he falls.

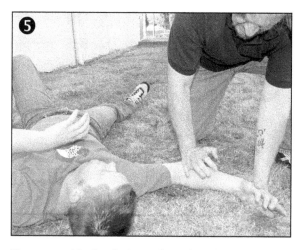

The moment he lands, brace it against the ground and hit the target again. Flee.

FINGERS: ACUTE PAIN TECHNIQUES

I place finger techniques into the acute pain category I talked about earlier. They were useful during the years I worked skid row, a place where 75 percent of the people I contacted were intoxicated, in advanced stages of alcoholism, and often violent.

I didn't know about pain sensors then so I labeled my techniques "general pain" and "acute pain." Still do. For example, I call a wristlock a general pain technique and I call bending the little finger back acute pain. When I would apply a standard wristlock on a guy and he just looked at me with a puzzled expression, I'd quickly grab one of his fingers and crank it in the direction it wasn't intended to go. Not only would he go up on his tiptoes in agony, he would admit to any and all crimes, like kidnapping the Lindbergh baby. This was because the acute pain technique better penetrates the dulled brain. While the words "general" and "acute" still apply, the real reason acute techniques work better has to do with the number and distribution of pain sensors in the targets, as well as the type of nerve conduction pathway traversed by electric signals coming from them.

Two Types of Pain

Scientists know that there are two types of pain: fast pain and slow. When one part of the body is traumatized, a pain receptor sends signals up to the brain via one of the fast or slow pathways. The fast pain pathway best serves our purposes in martial arts: It instantaneously gets an attacker's attention, and thus allows you to seize the moment.

KEY CONCEPT

In short, a wristlock doesn't activate the same number of pain sensors as does a finger technique. Therefore, consider twisting, bending and stretching the fingers as go-to moves when dealing with someone whose pain sensors are mildly dulled.

PINKIE JAM

You're trying to move a slightly resisting person a short distance with a wristlock when he begins to move his arm, clearly not feeling your technique (as much as he should) and on the verge of pulling away from you.

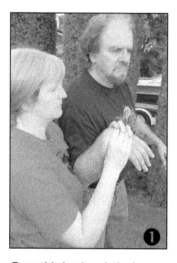

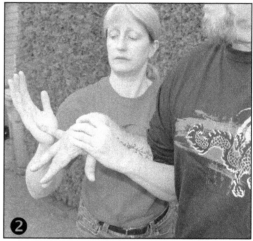

From this basic wristlock position....

...catch his finger with the heel of your hand...

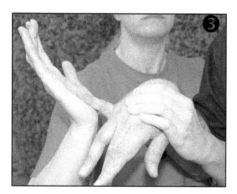

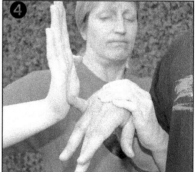

...and push it toward the back of his hand as far as it will go.

Then push it across his other fingers (it won't go that far). When he reacts to the more acute pain signals, you can walk him a short distance. If things deteriorate, you can jam his little finger as hard as you can to sprain or break it. Then flee.

THE SPLITS

You've already knocked a big guy's hands away twice.

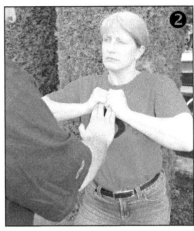

He puts his hands on your chest.

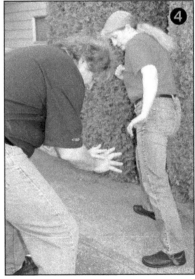

Grab two fingers with your left hand and two with your right.

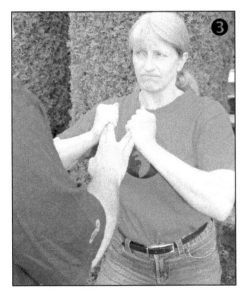

Split them down the middle. Pull them apart slowly as you verbalize your displeasure or yank them in opposite directions to destroy his ability to ever do it again.

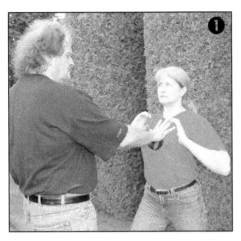

Flee as the acute agony penetrates his dulled brain.

FINGER BEND

The obnoxious drunk has pushed you several times. Don't try to grab his finger out of the air. Grab his wrist.

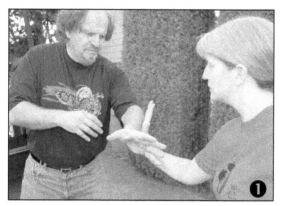

Swat his wrist to the side.

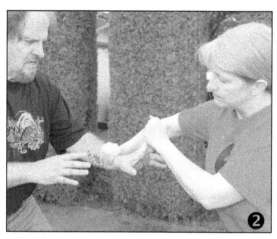

Grab it and quickly secure one or two fingers.

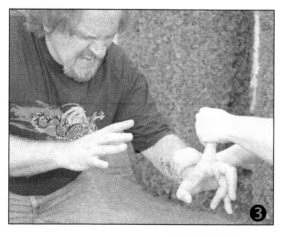

The wrist grab creates a solid base as you ram his finger back.

Options:

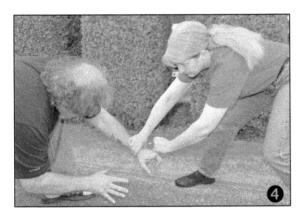

Option 1:
When he bends forward in an attempt to relive the pain, continue to push downward to...

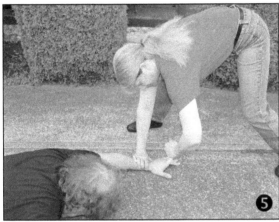

... force him to the ground.

Option 2:
Instead of taking him down, ram his finger toward the back of his hand to hyperextend or even break the joint. Then flee.

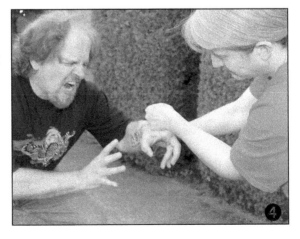

CHAPTER 9

LEGS: FEMORAL NERVE, KNEES & PERONEAL NERVE

It's faster to bring down a tree by chopping its trunk than by picking its leaves. The same is true of an attacker's "trunk." When his legs are inadvertently presented to you, here are a few targets that when struck have a crippling effect, even on a person impervious to pain.

FEMORAL NERVE

This is a great target that activates the somatic reflex arc discussed in Chapter 6. This means that when the nerve is struck or pressed sharply, the attacker will jerk forward a little or a lot, a moment when you should flee or take him down.

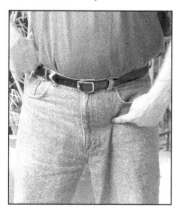

The femoral nerves are found at the top of both thighs in the crease where they attach to the pelvis, three or four inches over from the groin. (Free tip: To remember where it is, walk around pointing at yours and other people's for three days.)

FOOT PUSH

You don't have to kick the target to get the effect. Just push it sharply.

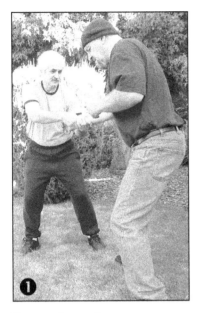 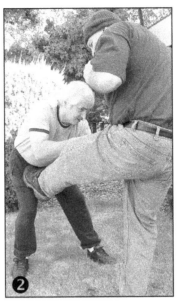

The attacker grabs your arm.

Quickly ram your foot into his femoral nerve.

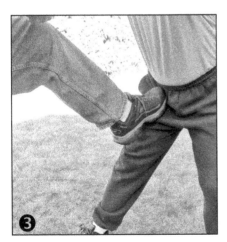 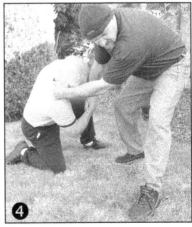

Press in with a forceful thrust as you yank his arm toward you. If you can't yank his arm, at least solidify it so more force goes into the target.

When he jackknifes forward, pull him to the ground by his hair, collar or head.

HAND PRESS

You're clinching for dominance. As always, you're looking for a window of opportunity to make your move.

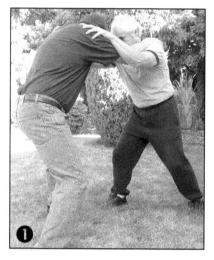

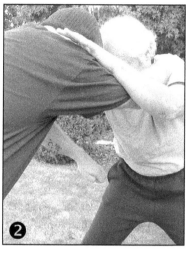

There is a sudden weakness in his right arm while his right leg is forward.

Sharply ram your middle knuckles...

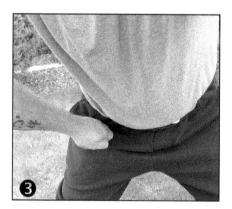

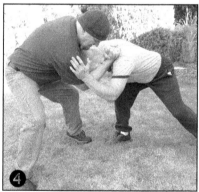

...into his right femoral nerve. Be alert because sometimes people jerk forward so forcefully that you might bang heads.

Pull him forward and down to the ground.

KNEES

On cold days I walk with a limp, a not so subtle reminder of breaking my knee in 1975. I've written in other books about my long recovery so I'll refrain from telling the story here. I will say, however, that a broken knee holds a secure first place on the pain scale of "What hurts the most." Second place is diving head first into a wood chipper.

We've all heard people say that it takes about 14 pounds of impact to break a knee; depending on the speaker it might be more or less. I really don't know because I've never seen one broken from a kick, nor have any of my buddies in the fighting arts. Mine was fractured from a twist. However, it's common for people to be disabled briefly when accidentally kicked in the knee in training or deliberately kicked there in a real fight.

Although a kick to the knee can be extraordinarily painful, we're dealing with people who won't feel it, or not much. Therefore, you must think in terms of debilitating the attacker, regardless of whether he feels anything.

There are many ways to attack the knee. Here are two.

AN INCH OR SO ABOVE THE KNEECAP

The first target is a nerve strike that works rather like poking the delete button on your keyboard. Just as you don't have to poke "Delete" hard to make your typing disappear, it takes only a medium-force kick just above the knee cap to make the leg seemingly

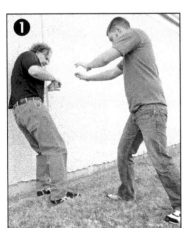

disappear and leave the rest of the body to crash to the ground.

It's not an easy target to hit since it's a small area, but when you can nail it, the rewards are immediate. Although any kick will work, let's use a sidekick and think of it as striking with the blade of an axe.

The attacker has pushed you against something and now he's advancing.

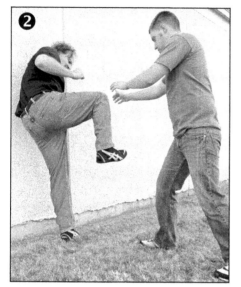

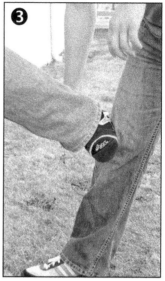

Drive a sidekick...

...into his leg an inch or two above his kneecap.

When his leg starts to collapse, push him down.

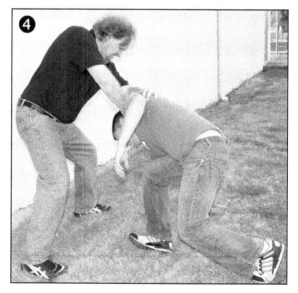

DAMAGE THE KNEE

In this situation, your objective is to cause so much damage to the knee joint that the attacker can no longer function. I would argue that while the knee cap is quite vulnerable, it still requires sufficient damage to put it out of commission. In other words, it would behoove you to have good power and speed as part of your arsenal. Also, you want to create or take advantage of moments when the knee will not give with your blow.

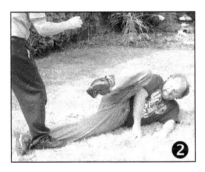

You're down and the attacker comes after you.

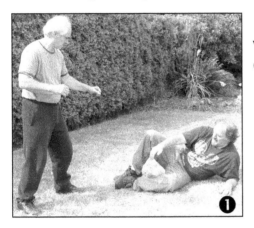

To prevent his leg from moving with your kick, hook your foot behind his closest one. Chamber your upper leg...

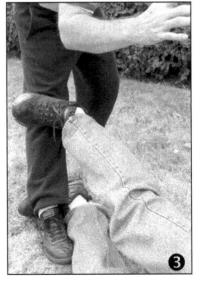

...and smash his knee with the heel half of your foot.

SMASH BRACED KNEE

Anytime the knee is supported by Mother Earth (or Mother Sidewalk) is a good time to stomp it. Aim an inch above the kneecap and follow with another stomp directly onto the kneecap. That way you impact the nerve point and damage the structure.

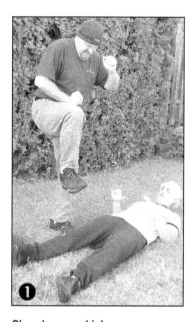

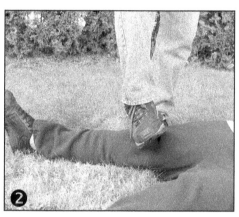

Stomp the nerve point an inch above his knee cap.

Chamber your kick.

Option:

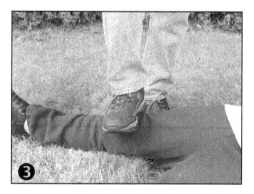

Stomp his kneecap as an initial technique or as a follow-up to the nerve stomp.

PERONEAL NERVE

Imagine that you're wearing pants with a stripe down the outside of each pant leg. That is roughly the path that the peroneal nerve takes from your hip to the side of your knee. It extends farther down but it's the upper leg that we're interested in. Now separate this pathway into three sections. The area most vulnerable to impact (measuring from the hip down) is where the first section ends and the second begins. From a standing position, hit it with an upper angle kick, a horizontal kick, or a slightly downward one. Some fighters prefer one angle over the other, but they are all good.

If you have been kicked in the peroneal you know it begets pain and nausea. You either had trouble standing or you spiraled to the floor. Pain resistant people might not feel it, but the blow almost always has a debilitating effect. There will also be some degree of somatic reflex arc, in that the attacker's upper body will fold in the direction of the struck leg. This gives you the option of moving in quickly to execute a takedown in the direction he's leaning.

Here are a few short scenarios in which you can hit the peroneal.

CLINCH

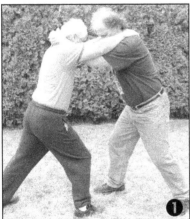

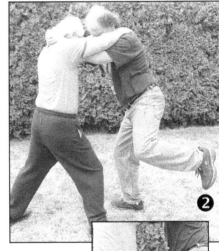

When the moment is right... and you can lift your leg, ram your knee into the attacker's peroneal.

AGAINST A PUSH

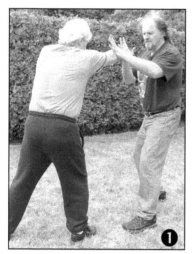

Knock his arms aside.

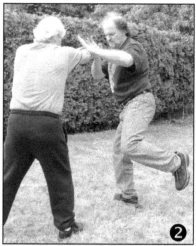

Whip an upper roundhouse...

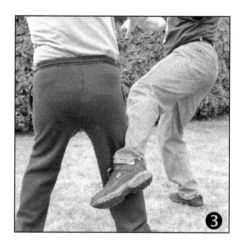

...into his peroneal. Hit with your shin.

PUNCH IT

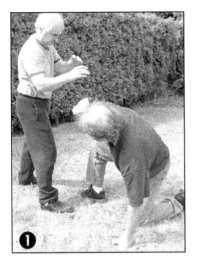

You're down, he's up...

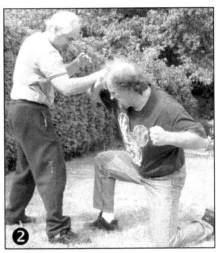

...and moving in. Cover your head...

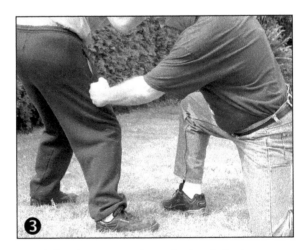

...and slam in a peroneal punch when he's close.
Don't snap it; punch deeply.

STOMP IT

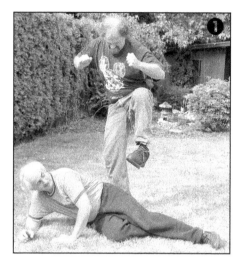

He's down and you're up. To keep him down...

...stomp down onto his braced peroneal. (I once accidentally hit a fellow trainer in a police defensive class in this position and he missed several days of work. Yes, he was mad.)

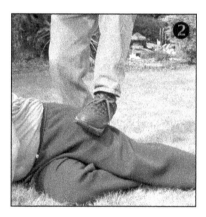

CHAPTER 10

TAKEDOWNS

A powerful option for dealing with people who are impervious to pain is to unbalance them and send them on a crash course to the sidewalk.

WHY TAKE 'EM DOWN?

When that assailant grins after you groin kick him, he looks questioningly at you after you punch him in the ribs, and he snickers when you palm-heel his chin, it's time to dump him. Here's why:

- Effective takedowns are based on the loss of balance not pain.
- There are fewer ways for him to attack you from the ground.
- A hard landing might disorient him.
- Targets that are supported by the floor are often more debilitating.
- Taking the aggressor down allows you to escape.

Before I comment on each of these, let me remind you that there are no absolutes and no guarantees with any of these bullets because there are no guarantees whenever you deal with the human condition. Never is this truer than when the adversary is impervious to pain.

Effective takedowns are based on the loss of balance not pain

Everyone, no matter what their state of mind, is susceptible to going down when their balance is taken away.

There are fewer ways for him to attack you from the ground

A standing attacker is free to move in any direction he chooses. Add to this freedom his ability to withstand your pain techniques and you have a highly dangerous situation. If you're unable to attack any of the debilitating targets discussed in this book, dumping the adversary onto the ground is a solid tactical move that reduces his mobility and the number of ways he can attack.

A hard landing might disorient him

Emphasis on the word *might*. If he can tolerate pain when he is standing, a spine-jarring slam and a skull-cracking thump against cement might not stop his aggression either. Then again, it might, as it depends on what part of his head hits. His natural fear of falling and a hard landing might bring him back to reality and make him easier to control. Or it might not.

Targets that are supported by the floor are often more debilitating

When a target is supported, all of the blow's kinetic energy goes into it. When you stomp an attacker's vital points—forearm, outer thigh—close to 100 percent of the blow's energy goes into the unyielding target.

Taking the aggressor down allows you to escape

Fights are all about opportunities, moments as brief as a slightly dropped lead-hand guard, or as long as a few seconds bought when the attacker is dazed by a hard slam to the ground.

The law prefers that you flee a fight when you have the opportunity rather than remain at the scene to continue brawling. A savvy lawyer for the attacker will ask if you had an opportunity to escape. If you did but didn't take it, he will make you the bad guy. Or should you *over*-defend yourself and beat the attacker senseless, the district attorney might go after you for continuing to fight when you had an opportunity to get away.

Should the attacker back you into a corner and your best defensive blows go unnoticed by him, look for that open window, take him down, and then run like the wind. Fleeing will prevent him from hurting you and the sometimes crazy legal system from blaming you.

BALANCE AND UNBALANCING MADE SIMPLE

Too many martial artists seem to go out of their way to make techniques, concepts and principles complex. Why? Why convolute something that should be simple, direct and to the point? Why confuse things with complicated jargon and mystical explanations? Although volumes have been written on the subject of balance, here is a short explanation, a simple approach that has always worked for me.

TRIPOD CONCEPT

A camera tripod doesn't fall over because it has three legs to keep it upright. As a two-legged animal, you don't fall over into a pile because you have something called equilibrium that works to keep you upright. Nonetheless, your balance is still somewhat vulnerable in the direction where that third leg would be if you were a tripod.

Stand up and spread your feet three feet apart. Look down and find the spot half way between your two feet (it will be straight down from your navel, unless your belly button is off center). Now look 12 to 18 inches out in front of you from that center spot. That is where your balance is weakest. You're also vulnerable 12 to 18 inches out behind you from that same center. No matter how you configure your feet, imagine where that third leg would be if you were a tripod. That is where your balance is weakest.

There are zillions of takedowns in the grappling arts and most are effective against a pain-resistant attacker. Once you upset his balance to start him on a journey to the ground, it doesn't matter how intoxicated, mentally ill or angry he is.

Here are a few simple takedowns that have worked for my martial arts friends and me. Let's start at the head and work our way down to the legs.

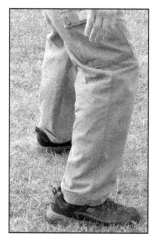
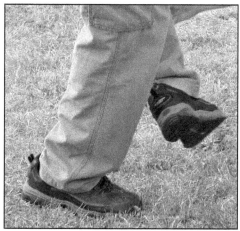

No matter what the foot configuration, the attacker is off balance when pushed or pulled in the direction of where his third support leg would be.

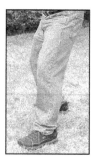
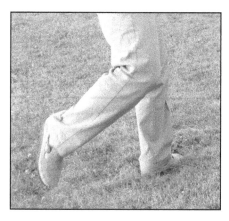

EASY TAKEDOWNS

HAIR PULL

All of the head techniques here apply the old axiom "where the head goes the body follows." Never is this truer than when pulling an attacker's hair downward, or in any direction for that matter. I've written a lot about hair techniques because I've used them often when dealing with violent people. There are two key elements that apply here.

- The pain can be acute, depending on how you pull the hair, from which part of the head you pull it, and the recipient's ability to tolerate it.
- Since you're applying the technique at the highest point of the attacker's body, you're in a good position to control where and how hard he falls.

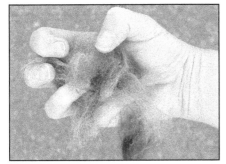

Hair techniques can get ugly.

The attacker tries to grab you.

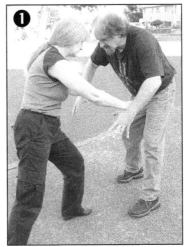

Block his drunken two-handed push.

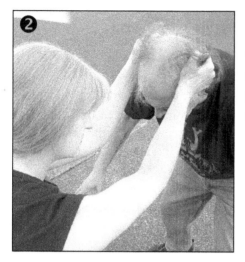

Thrust your hands deep into the hair at the sides of his head and make a fist against his scalp.

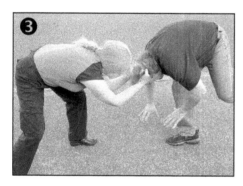

Jerk his head downward in the direction of that invisible tripod leg.

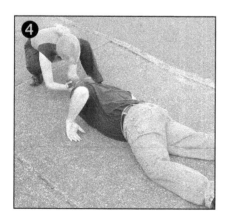

Step back to give him a place to fall. Hold his head down by rotating your fisted hands toward you.

Option:

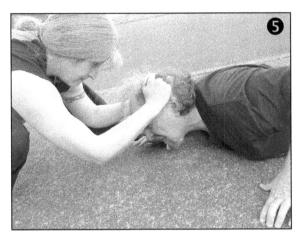

Should he lift his head to get up (don't let him up any farther than pictured)...

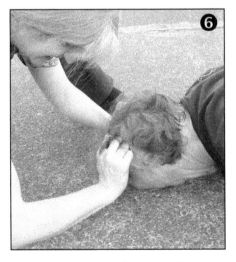

...slam his face, nose first, into the pavement to stun him and activate his tears.

THE STUMBLING ATTACKER

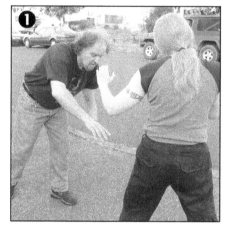

The drunken attacker loses his balance as he lunges.

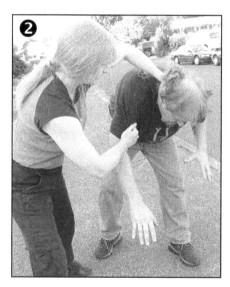

Sidestep and grab his upper arm or sleeve, and a wad of hair at the back of his head. Lift your elbow for strength...

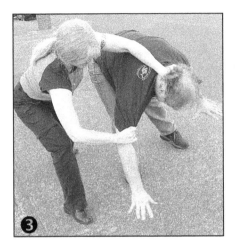

...and push his head forward and down toward his invisible tripod leg as you pull his arm in the same direction.

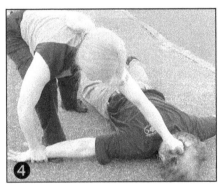

Once he's prone, continue to rip his hair forward to jam his face into the pavement as you rotate his hand upward to lock his elbow.

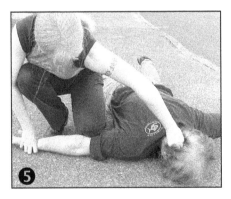

Lean your knee on his ulna nerve one inch above his elbow. Although, he might not feel the pain, the primary purpose is to use this leverage point as well as the hair technique to keep him pinned to the street. Wait for help to arrive or flee when you can.

FOREHEAD PUSH

Here is an example of the axiom: "The best defense is a good offense." While drunks and dopers might have slow reflexes, the mentally deranged, the enraged or the overly-large person might be as quick as a cat. Never underestimate your adversary. Choose the moment wisely.

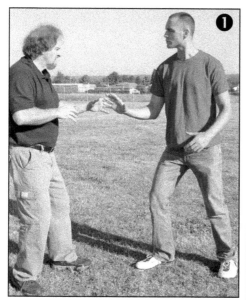 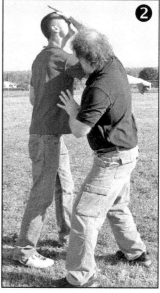

He threatens by words and body language. Swat his arm aside and...

...move outside of it. Slap your palm against his forehead.

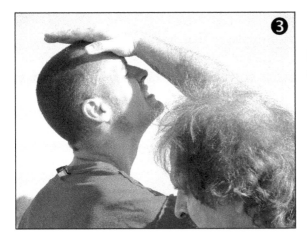

Push his face up to
disorient him...

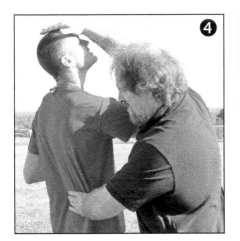

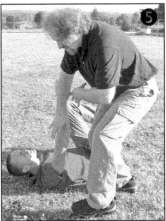

...as you begin to walk quickly past his
side. Usually pushing the forehead up
and over is enough to take him down,
but if he suddenly balks, push on the
small of his back with your other hand.
The key is to keep walking as you do
this...

...until he crashes to Mother
Earth. Flee the scene.

FACE GRAB AND PUSH

The concept here is similar to "Forehead push" except you're grabbing the attacker's face and covering his eyes, which can have an even greater disorientation effect as the head is being pushed up and over. Here is an offensive approach.

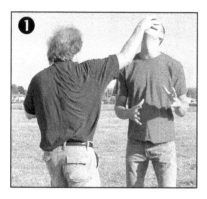

The attacker threatens. Act preemptively by grabbing his face.

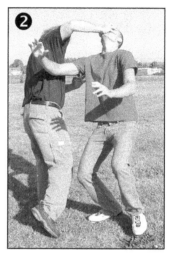

As you move forward and past him...

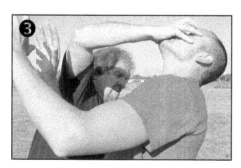

...push his face up and over...

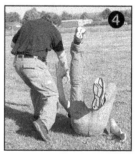

...in the direction of his invisible third leg until he falls onto his back.

PHILTRUM PUSH

This is a favorite of my friend Rory Miller, a former corrections officer and author of *Meditations on Violence*. Rory, who calls it "spine extension" because of the stress it places on the recipient's back, has used this against really big men as well as people high on PCP and other pain-numbing drugs. You can use any of the entries from "Forehead push," "Face Grab and Push," and "Neck Hook." Or:

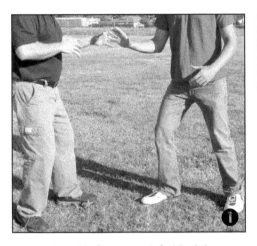

Try to mirror his feet—your left, his right—so you don't have to cross step.

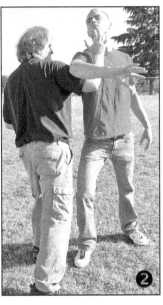

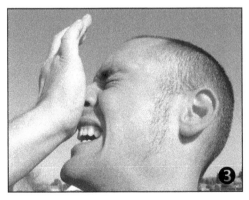

Move when his mind is occupied with talking or listening to you. Lunge step or drop step just past his right side. Swat his reaching arm aside, or do as shown, and step just outside his reach as you shoot your hand under his arm and toward his face. You can probably go over the top of his arm if you're a lot taller than him.

As you bring up your rear foot to solidify your base, slam your palm under his chin or against his philtrum. Both are good points to push so the body easily follows. The philtrum is an especially good leverage point though the risk of getting bit is a tad higher.

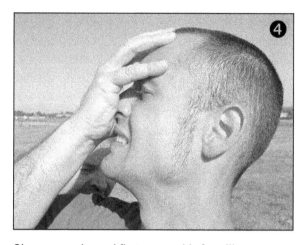

Glom your palm and fingers over his face like an octopus.

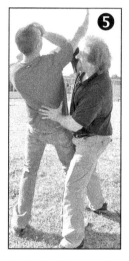

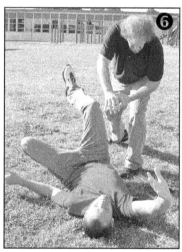

The instant you make contact, push his face up and over as your other palm presses against his spine just above his hips.

Down he goes. Flee.

NECK HOOK

As the name implies, your arm forms a hook in which you catch the attacker's neck. This is as low as you can go and still apply the principle of "where the head goes the body follows." Depending on the situation, either place your arm around his neck or whip it around his throat with great force. Be justified to use the latter.

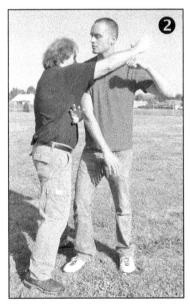

Swat the attacker's reaching arms aside and...

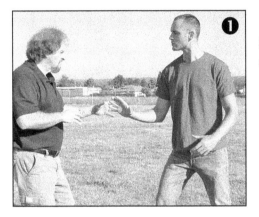

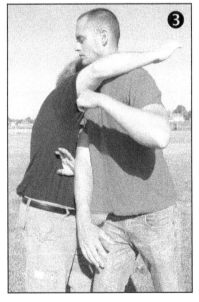

...keep pressing his closest arm across his body as you lunge forward and shoot your other arm up...

...and around his neck. I like to point with my fingers believing it helps to project energy in my hand and arm in the direction of his invisible third leg.

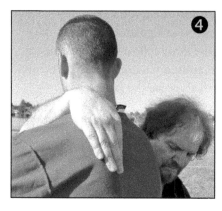

Don't drape your hand over his shoulder. This stops your energy at his shoulder.

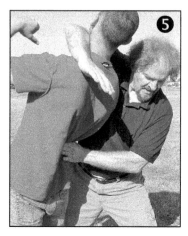

Place your other hand on his closest love handle just above his hip and lift your hooking elbow to begin tilting his world.

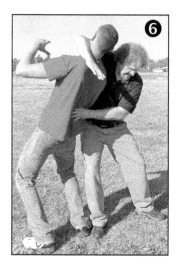

Push on his love handle as you continue lifting his chin. As he begins to fall toward his invisible third leg, use your hooking arm to twist his upper body counter clockwise toward you as you pull his love handle toward you. Take a small step to the...

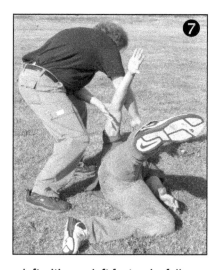

...left with your left foot so he falls down in front of you.

TWIST, HIT AND PULL

This is a favorite of my friend Shawn Kovacich, author of the excellent multi-book series *Achieving Kicking Excellence*. Shawn used this move when he worked as a bouncer in some tough beer joints where many of the patrons were "feeling no pain." Shawn would set up his technique with a rainstorm of palm-heel strikes to jar and confuse the attacker's pain-resistant brain.

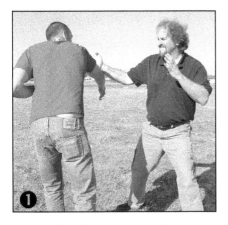

You knock aside the attacker's arm with your right hand.

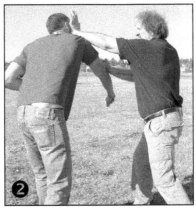

Ram a palm-heel strike into his jawbone to discombobulate his thinking.

Chamber quickly and...

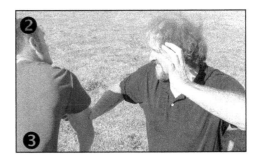

...hit him again. Although he isn't feeling pain, multiple hits should stun him.

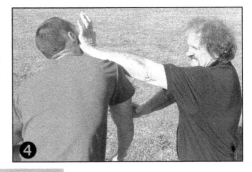

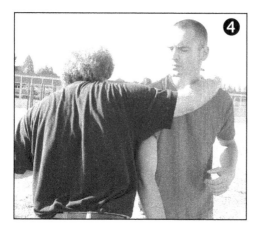

Move quickly behind him as you slip your arm around his neck to gain leverage and reduce his ability to breathe. You now have options as to what you can do.

Options:

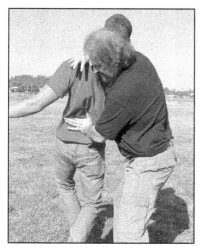

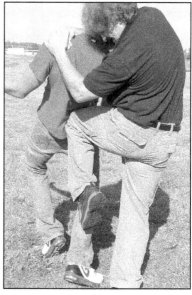

Option 1: Force him backwards by pressing your hand into his lower back. Continue to press until he falls.

Option 2: Ram your knee into a kidney to quickly weaken him and then pull him to the ground.

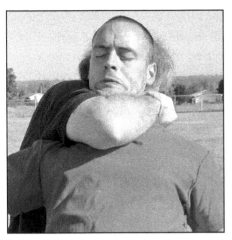 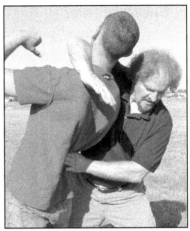

Option 3: Apply a carotid constraint (see Chapter 5 as to how to lower him).

Option 4: To walk him backwards out of a bar or party, elevate your elbow to lift his chin. This gives him direction and removes your arm from his throat, a location where excessive pressure from pulling him could cause internal injury.

Bend Him Backwards

Forcing an attacker over backwards places him virtually under your control. It's a great position to maneuver a pain-resistant attacker since it's not predicated on pain, but rather leverage and gravity. It's a position in which he suddenly becomes weak with few defensive options, while you become strong with many.

Should he somehow maneuver himself so that you begin to lose the advantage, immediately apply a takedown technique of your choice.

KEY CONCEPT

Shoulder Twist

Here is the ol' push and pull shoulder twist used in earlier techniques. I'm using it again because it's a great way to set up a variety of takedowns against a pain-resistant attacker. Execute it anytime a window of opportunity opens to get behind him.

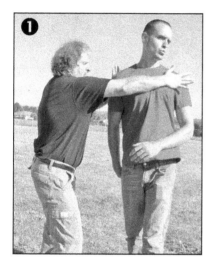

Lunge forward and push the farthest shoulder and pull the closest.

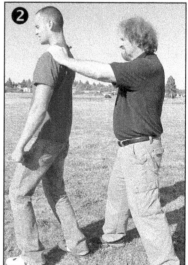

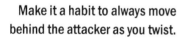

Make it a habit to always move behind the attacker as you twist.

There are lots of ways to get him down now. Here are three of my favorites:

FOREHEAD PULL:

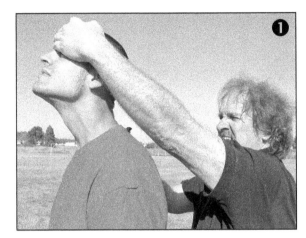

Reach up and over to palm his forehead.

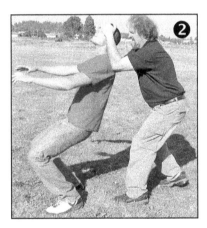

Tuck your elbow to create downward energy.

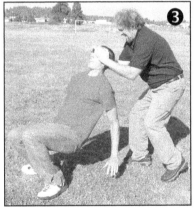

Pull his head back and downward toward his invisible third leg.

LOCK KNEES AND PUSH:

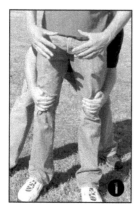

Slap your palms around his knees.

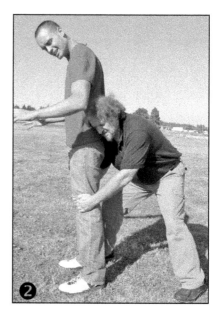

Hold them tightly as you press his butt with your shoulder. This will lock his knees or nearly lock them.

Down he goes. Know that some people, because of their mental state, might not catch themselves with their hands.

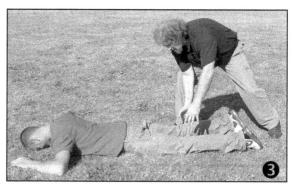

Leg pop takedown:

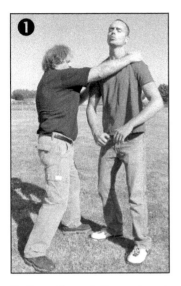

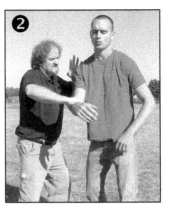

...grab his upper arm and...

Half way through the push and pull...

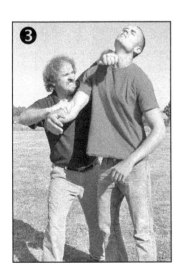

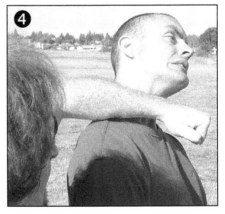

...shoot your other forearm against the side of his neck to...

...strike his brachial plexus. This will stun him for a moment as you use your forearm to push against his neck to assist in the takedown.

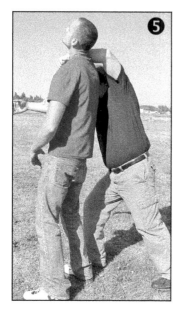

Slam your thigh...

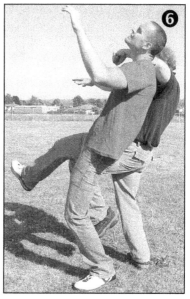

...against the back of his leg as you push his head back.

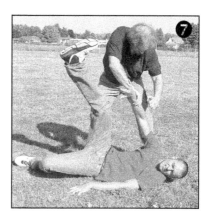

Down he goes.

BODY TAKEDOWN

I learned this from Mark Mireles, with whom I coauthored *Fighting in the Clinch* and *Street Stoppers*. By trapping one of the attacker's arms, you can slam his pinned side into walls and cars, or take him to the ground on that side so he can't catch himself.

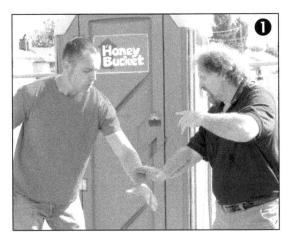

The attacker reaches or punches toward you. Block his arm toward the inside of his body far enough that you're able to easily...

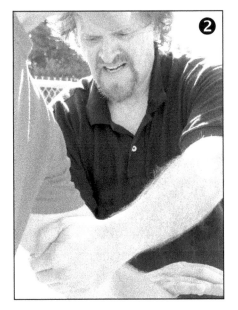

...grab his upper arm. Use a thumbless grip—press your thumb tightly against your index finger—to prevent injury to your thumb should he flail his arm.

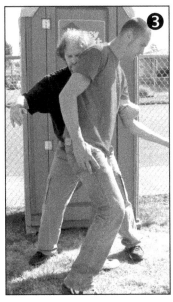

Step behind him quickly and...

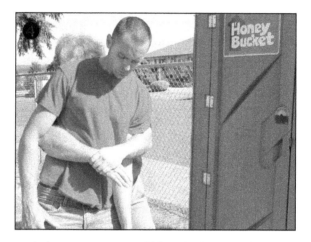

...circle your arms around him, pinning his left. Clasp hands. Take him to the ground in the direction of his pinned arm or...

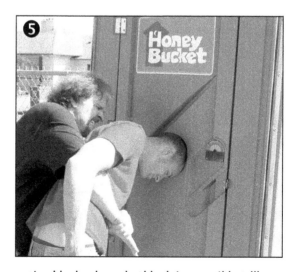

...stun him by slamming him into something, like an outhouse.

LEG TAKEDOWNS

There are many leg takedowns that are good against a person impervious to pain. One that I've used the most is the good ol' osoto geri, a leg sweep technique I first learned from a book in the 1950s when I was in grade school. I memorized it and then tried it out on the playground. Two things happened: It worked like a charm and I got sent to the principal's office.

I like that the technique is forgiving. That is, it almost always works even when you do a poor job of execution.

Here are my two favorite variations.

FACE SMOTHER AND LEG SWEEP

The aforementioned face smother adds disorientation to the hard landing.

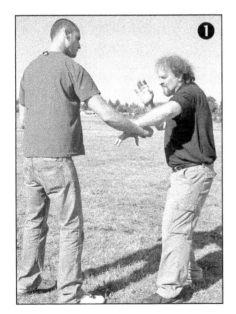 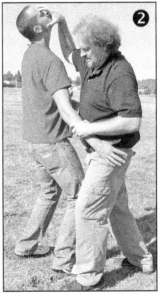

Block the attacker's reach.

Step forward, placing your foot about eight inches away from his foot, and angled outward about 45 degrees. Smack your open hand over...

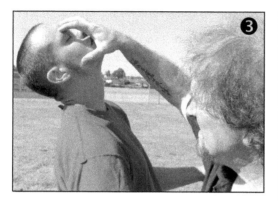

...the attacker's face.

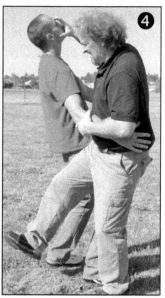

Pull his arm down as you push his face up and over. Swing your leg past him...

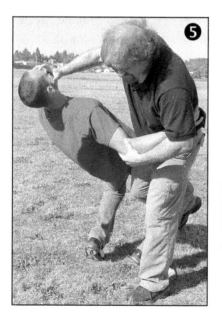

... and bring it back against the back of his leg.

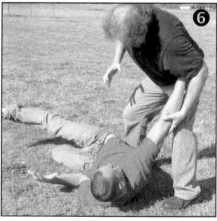

Take him down at about a 45-degree angle, which makes it hard for him to resist. Flee.

BACK GRIP AND LEG SWEEP

This arguably works best when you grip the attacker at upper center, as pictured here, though pulling at mid back sometimes work, too. It depends on the size and strength of the attacker, and the direction of his energy. If you got a choice, go for upper center.

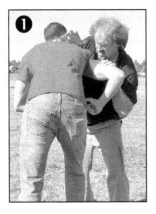

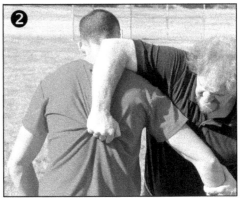

The assailant tries a sloppy clinch. Shoot your hand over his shoulder, clipping his jaw with your forearm to snap his head back. This starts his energy moving back.

Grab his arm and a fist full of his shirt at the center of his upper back. The two of you are shoulder to shoulder at this point.

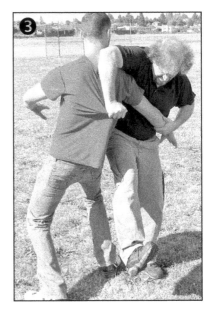

Whip your sweeping leg forward...

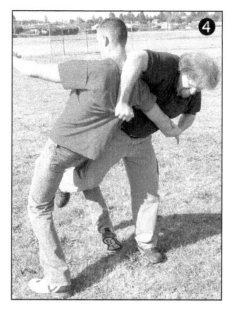

...and then back against his leg as you
drive your fist downward.

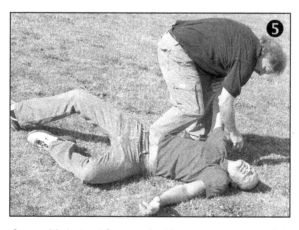

Sweep his leg out from under him as you ram your fist
toward the ground.

Note: Although the hits to the face in both of these variations
probably won't hurt the assailant, the blows force his energy and
balance in the direction you want him to go.

WARNING: "GROUND-AND-POUND"

Let's say you defend against an attacker with a hard roundhouse kick to the peroneal nerve on the outside of his thigh, which sends him to the floor, stunned and helpless. Then you take advantage of his grogginess and inability to fight by unleashing on him a hail storm of punches and kicks. Understand that this places you at risk of being charged criminally with using force that was unnecessary and unreasonable.

A savvy prosecuting attorney will likely bring up the mixed martial arts term, "ground-and-pound," a popular phrase used in competition to describe the repeated striking of a downed opponent by one who is in the dominate position. The striking continues until the referee stops it. A prosecutor might argue that your actions define ground-and-pound, and that you were brutally out of control.

Here is how to avoid being snagged by this term:

- Use only necessary and reasonable force when acting in self-defense.
- Keep "ground and pound" out of your vocabulary, even if you're a competitor.
- Be prepared to explain how the term does not describe *your* personal code of self-defense and training philosophy.
- Be ready to explain that your force was based on the action/reaction format. "The attacker assaulted me [the act] and I responded in self-defense [the reaction]. I continued to defend myself until I had an opportunity to run (or get the attacker under control)."

Save yourself a lot of money and grief by training to get away from the attacker after he has been stunned. Untangle yourself, scoot away from him, get up, and flee. Or if the situation is such that you need to restrain him, do so using a technique that relies on leverage instead of pain.

Take it from a guy who has seen many lives ruined by a burst of temper, a ridiculous need for payback, or a final cheap shot. Don't do it.

Resist the desire and live a hassle-free life.

CONCLUSION

Self-defense is more than reacting quickly to a sudden threat; it's also about preplanning, and understanding the incredible frailties and resiliencies of the human body. Some people drop from what appears to be a minor assault, while others withstand unbelievable punishment. It's this last group that we have addressed in this book and the type of attacker that you must think about in advance.

I began training in the martial arts in the 1960s, a time when fighters were convinced that their techniques were so deadly that all they had to do was kick or punch an assailant anywhere on their body and the person would go down. Many still believe this.

Similarly, there has been a long-time debate among gun enthusiasts as to which caliber of bullet is the most lethal. I've always responded to this by asking, "Would you rather get shot in the leg with a .45 or in the heart with a .22? Or, as one writer noted on a firearms blog: "It's not what you throw at 'em; it's where you hit 'em. Just ask David (of David and Goliath)."

Just as many martial artists are convinced that they possess fight-stopping punches, kicks and throws, too many cops think that a bullet will end a situation. Here are a few incidents that surprised my fellow officers:

- In two different situations—a male in one and a female in the other—were shot in the head five times by their spouses. Five skull-smashing bullets in each victim and both lived, one even fought with the responding officers.

- A police buddy was disarmed of his baton by a suspect who then commenced to beat the officer with it. During the struggle, the officer managed to fire one round that punched through the assailant's heart. Although the bullet would kill him 90 seconds later, the man continued to beat the officer for several more seconds before he turned and ran. The assailant died in mid stride a few yards away.
- I once fought an extraordinarily combative hold-up man inside of an ambulance just minutes after he had been shot by another officer. The bullet destroyed the suspect's lower spine and subsequently made him a paraplegic. I eventually got him controlled using a sleeper hold.
- Two officers confronted a man under the influence of PCP. The suspect immediately killed one of them and commenced beating the other. That officer managed to empty his gun into the man, though the man was unfazed and continued to fight. Somehow the officer reloaded, and when another round struck the man's pelvic bowl, breaking it where it connects with the head of his femur (thigh bone), he finally collapsed to the sidewalk. The officer quickly scooted away a few steps, but the nightmare wasn't over. The crumpled and mortally wounded man began to crawl toward the officer, killing etched on his face, blood spurting from his many wounds. He continued to crawl until his veins and arteries ran empty and his dying heart pumped only air.

Just as the police were shocked to see these assailant's shattered by bullets but continue to fight with ferocity, many martial artists have been dumbfounded to see their attackers shake off their punches and kicks. Although bullets are clearly more lethal than martial arts techniques, what they share in common is that they both require precise target selection to stop a threat that is impervious to pain.

As I've preached for years in my books and DVDs, there are no guarantees in a fight for survival, and never is that more true than when facing an attacker who is impervious to pain. However, you increase your odds of winning when you understand how the human brain functions under certain conditions, when you understand how the body's pain receptors work, and when you know which targets, that when struck, debilitate without relying on the brain receiving pain signals.

I hope this book begins your understanding of this critical information.

Train hard

Loren W. Christensen
Portland, Oregon

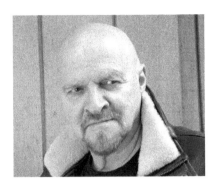

ABOUT THE AUTHOR

Loren W. Christensen is a Vietnam veteran and retired police officer with 29 years of law enforcement experience.

As a martial arts student and teacher since 1965, he has earned an 8th dan in American Free Style Karate, a 2nd dan in aiki jujitsu, and a 1st dan in Modern Arnis. He has starred in seven instructional martial arts DVDs. In 2011, Loren was inducted into the Masters Hall of Fame, garnering the Golden Lifetime Achievement Award.

As a writer, Loren has worked with five publishers, penning over 50 books, nonfiction and fiction on a variety of subjects. His thriller fiction series *Dukkha* is popular among martial artists. He has written dozens of magazine articles on a variety of topics to include, martial arts, nutrition, bodybuilding, police tactics, survival skills, meditation, and mental imagery.

He can be contacted through his website at www.lwcbooks.com.

BOOKS FROM YMAA

6 HEALING MOVEMENTS
101 REFLECTIONS ON TAI CHI CHUAN
108 INSIGHTS INTO TAI CHI CHUAN
ADVANCING IN TAE KWON DO
ANALYSIS OF SHAOLIN CHIN NA 2ND ED
ANCIENT CHINESE WEAPONS
ART OF HOJO UNDO
ARTHRITIS RELIEF, 3RD ED.
BACK PAIN RELIEF, 2ND ED.
BAGUAZHANG, 2ND ED.
CARDIO KICKBOXING ELITE
CHIN NA IN GROUND FIGHTING
CHINESE FAST WRESTLING
CHINESE FITNESS
CHINESE TUI NA MASSAGE
CHOJUN
COMPREHENSIVE APPLICATIONS OF SHAOLIN
      CHIN NA
CONFLICT COMMUNICATION
CROCODILE AND THE CRANE: A NOVEL
CUTTING SEASON: A XENON PEARL MARTIAL ARTS
      THRILLER
DEFENSIVE TACTICS
DESHI: A CONNOR BURKE MARTIAL ARTS THRILLER
DIRTY GROUND
DR. WU'S HEAD MASSAGE
DUKKHA HUNGRY GHOSTS
DUKKHA REVERB
DUKKHA, THE SUFFERING: AN EYE FOR AN EYE
DUKKHA UNLOADED
ENZAN: THE FAR MOUNTAIN, A CONNOR BURKE MARTIAL
      ARTS THRILLER
ESSENCE OF SHAOLIN WHITE CRANE
EXPLORING TAI CHI
FACING VIOLENCE
FIGHT BACK
FIGHT LIKE A PHYSICIST
THE FIGHTER'S BODY
FIGHTER'S FACT BOOK
FIGHTER'S FACT BOOK 2
FIGHTING THE PAIN RESISTANT ATTACKER
FIRST DEFENSE
FORCE DECISIONS: A CITIZENS GUIDE
FOX BORROWS THE TIGER'S AWE
INSIDE TAI CHI
KAGE: THE SHADOW, A CONNOR BURKE MARTIAL ARTS
      THRILLER
KATA AND THE TRANSMISSION OF KNOWLEDGE
KRAV MAGA PROFESSIONAL TACTICS
KRAV MAGA WEAPON DEFENSES
LITTLE BLACK BOOK OF VIOLENCE
LIUHEBAFA FIVE CHARACTER SECRETS
MARTIAL ARTS ATHLETE
MARTIAL ARTS INSTRUCTION
MARTIAL WAY AND ITS VIRTUES
MASK OF THE KING
MEDITATIONS ON VIOLENCE
MIND/BODY FITNESS
THE MIND INSIDE TAI CHI
THE MIND INSIDE YANG STYLE TAI CHI CHUAN
MUGAI RYU
NATURAL HEALING WITH QIGONG
NORTHERN SHAOLIN SWORD, 2ND ED.
OKINAWA'S COMPLETE KARATE SYSTEM: ISSHIN RYU
POWER BODY
PRINCIPLES OF TRADITIONAL CHINESE MEDICINE
QIGONG FOR HEALTH & MARTIAL ARTS 2ND ED.

QIGONG FOR LIVING
QIGONG FOR TREATING COMMON AILMENTS
QIGONG MASSAGE
QIGONG MEDITATION: EMBRYONIC BREATHING
QIGONG MEDITATION: SMALL CIRCULATION
QIGONG, THE SECRET OF YOUTH: DA MO'S CLASSICS
QUIET TEACHER: A XENON PEARL MARTIAL ARTS THRILLER
RAVEN'S WARRIOR
REDEMPTION
ROOT OF CHINESE QIGONG, 2ND ED.
SCALING FORCE
SENSEI: A CONNOR BURKE MARTIAL ARTS THRILLER
SHIHAN TE: THE BUNKAI OF KATA
SHIN GI TAI: KARATE TRAINING FOR BODY, MIND, AND
      SPIRIT
SIMPLE CHINESE MEDICINE
SIMPLE QIGONG EXERCISES FOR HEALTH, 3RD ED.
SIMPLIFIED TAI CHI CHUAN, 2ND ED.
SIMPLIFIED TAI CHI FOR BEGINNERS
SOLO TRAINING
SOLO TRAINING 2
SUDDEN DAWN: THE EPIC JOURNEY OF BODHIDHARMA
SUNRISE TAI CHI
SUNSET TAI CHI
SURVIVING ARMED ASSAULTS
TAE KWON DO: THE KOREAN MARTIAL ART
TAEKWONDO BLACK BELT POOMSAE
TAEKWONDO: A PATH TO EXCELLENCE
TAEKWONDO: ANCIENT WISDOM FOR THE MODERN
      WARRIOR
TAEKWONDO: DEFENSES AGAINST WEAPONS
TAEKWONDO: SPIRIT AND PRACTICE
TAO OF BIOENERGETICS
TAI CHI BALL QIGONG: FOR HEALTH AND MARTIAL ARTS
TAI CHI BALL WORKOUT FOR BEGINNERS
TAI CHI BOOK
TAI CHI CHIN NA: THE SEIZING ART OF TAI CHI CHUAN,
      2ND ED.
TAI CHI CHUAN CLASSICAL YANG STYLE, 2ND ED.
TAI CHI CHUAN MARTIAL APPLICATIONS
TAI CHI CHUAN MARTIAL POWER, 3RD ED.
TAI CHI CONNECTIONS
TAI CHI DYNAMICS
TAI CHI QIGONG, 3RD ED.
TAI CHI SECRETS OF THE ANCIENT MASTERS
TAI CHI SECRETS OF THE WU & LI STYLES
TAI CHI SECRETS OF THE WU STYLE
TAI CHI SECRETS OF THE YANG STYLE
TAI CHI SWORD: CLASSICAL YANG STYLE, 2ND ED.
TAI CHI SWORD FOR BEGINNERS
TAI CHI WALKING
TAIJIQUAN THEORY OF DR. YANG, JWING-MING
TENGU: THE MOUNTAIN GOBLIN, A CONNOR BURKE MAR-
      TIAL ARTS THRILLER
TIMING IN THE FIGHTING ARTS
TRADITIONAL CHINESE HEALTH SECRETS
TRADITIONAL TAEKWONDO

TRAINING FOR SUDDEN VIOLENCE
WAY OF KATA
WAY OF KENDO AND KENJITSU
WAY OF SANCHIN KATA
WAY TO BLACK BELT
WESTERN HERBS FOR MARTIAL ARTISTS
WILD GOOSE QIGONG
WOMAN'S QIGONG GUIDE
XINGYIQUAN

DVDS FROM YMAA

ADVANCED PRACTICAL CHIN NA IN-DEPTH

ANALYSIS OF SHAOLIN CHIN NA

ATTACK THE ATTACK

BAGUAZHANG: EMEI BAGUAZHANG

CHEN STYLE TAIJIQUAN

CHIN NA IN-DEPTH COURSES 1—4

CHIN NA IN-DEPTH COURSES 5—8

CHIN NA IN-DEPTH COURSES 9—12

FACING VIOLENCE: 7 THINGS A MARTIAL ARTIST MUST KNOW

FIVE ANIMAL SPORTS

JOINT LOCKS

KNIFE DEFENSE: TRADITIONAL TECHNIQUES AGAINST A DAGGER

KUNG FU BODY CONDITIONING 1

KUNG FU BODY CONDITIONING 2

KUNG FU FOR KIDS

KUNG FU FOR TEENS

INFIGHTING

LOGIC OF VIOLENCE

MERIDIAN QIGONG

NEIGONG FOR MARTIAL ARTS

NORTHERN SHAOLIN SWORD : SAN CAI JIAN, KUN WU JIAN, QI MEN JIAN

QIGONG MASSAGE

QIGONG FOR HEALING

QIGONG FOR LONGEVITY

QIGONG FOR WOMEN

SABER FUNDAMENTAL TRAINING

SAI TRAINING AND SEQUENCES

SANCHIN KATA: TRADITIONAL TRAINING FOR KARATE POWER

SHAOLIN KUNG FU FUNDAMENTAL TRAINING: COURSES 1 & 2

SHAOLIN LONG FIST KUNG FU: BASIC SEQUENCES

SHAOLIN LONG FIST KUNG FU: INTERMEDIATE SEQUENCES

SHAOLIN LONG FIST KUNG FU: ADVANCED SEQUENCES 1

SHAOLIN LONG FIST KUNG FU: ADVANCED SEQUENCES 2

SHAOLIN SABER: BASIC SEQUENCES

SHAOLIN STAFF: BASIC SEQUENCES

SHAOLIN WHITE CRANE GONG FU BASIC TRAINING: COURSES 1 & 2

SHAOLIN WHITE CRANE GONG FU BASIC TRAINING: COURSES 3 & 4

SHUAI JIAO: KUNG FU WRESTLING

SIMPLE QIGONG EXERCISES FOR ARTHRITIS RELIEF

SIMPLE QIGONG EXERCISES FOR BACK PAIN RELIEF

SIMPLIFIED TAI CHI CHUAN: 24 & 48 POSTURES

SIMPLIFIED TAI CHI FOR BEGINNERS 48

SUNRISE TAI CHI

SUNSET TAI CHI

SWORD: FUNDAMENTAL TRAINING

TAEKWONDO KORYO POOMSAE

TAI CHI BALL QIGONG: COURSES 1 & 2

TAI CHI BALL QIGONG: COURSES 3 & 4

TAI CHI BALL WORKOUT FOR BEGINNERS

TAI CHI CHUAN CLASSICAL YANG STYLE

TAI CHI CONNECTIONS

TAI CHI ENERGY PATTERNS

TAI CHI FIGHTING SET

TAI CHI PUSHING HANDS: COURSES 1 & 2

TAI CHI PUSHING HANDS: COURSES 3 & 4

TAI CHI SWORD: CLASSICAL YANG STYLE

TAI CHI SWORD FOR BEGINNERS

TAI CHI SYMBOL: YIN YANG STICKING HANDS

TAIJI & SHAOLIN STAFF: FUNDAMENTAL TRAINING

TAIJI CHIN NA IN-DEPTH

TAIJI 37 POSTURES MARTIAL APPLICATIONS

TAIJI SABER CLASSICAL YANG STYLE

TAIJI WRESTLING

TRAINING FOR SUDDEN VIOLENCE

UNDERSTANDING QIGONG 1: WHAT IS QI? • HUMAN QI CIRCULATORY SYSTEM

UNDERSTANDING QIGONG 2: KEY POINTS • QIGONG BREATHING

UNDERSTANDING QIGONG 3: EMBRYONIC BREATHING

UNDERSTANDING QIGONG 4: FOUR SEASONS QIGONG

UNDERSTANDING QIGONG 5: SMALL CIRCULATION

UNDERSTANDING QIGONG 6: MARTIAL QIGONG BREATHING

WHITE CRANE HARD & SOFT QIGONG

WUDANG KUNG FU: FUNDAMENTAL TRAINING

WUDANG SWORD

WUDANG TAIJIQUAN

XINGYIQUAN

YANG TAI CHI FOR BEGINNERS

YMAA 25 YEAR ANNIVERSARY DVD

more products available from . . .
YMAA Publication Center, Inc. 楊氏東方文化出版中心
1-800-669-8892 • info@ymaa.com • www.ymaa.com

Printed in the USA
CPSIA information can be obtained
at www.ICGtesting.com
JSHW012050140824
68134JS00035B/3367